Health Policy and Disease in Colonial and Postcolonial Hong Kong, 1841–2003

Besides looking at major outbreaks of diseases and how they were coped with – diseases such as malaria, smallpox, tuberculosis, plague, venereal disease, avian flu, and SARS – this book also examines how the successive government regimes in Hong Kong took action to prevent diseases and control potential threats to health. It shows how policies impacted the various Chinese and non-Chinese groups, and how policies were often formulated as a result of negotiations between these different groups. By considering developments over a long historical period, the book contrasts the different approaches in the periods of colonial rule, Japanese occupation, postwar reconstruction, transition to decolonization, and Hong Kong as Special Administrative Region within the People's Republic of China.

Ka-che Yip is a Professor Emeritus of the University of Maryland Baltimore County, USA.

Yuen-sang Leung is Professor of History, Dean of Arts and Director of the Institute of Chinese Studies at the Chinese University of Hong Kong, China.

Man-kong Wong is Director of the China Studies Programme and Associate Professor of History at Hong Kong Baptist University, China.

Routledge Studies in the Modern History of Asia

For a full list of titles in this series, please visit www.routledge.com.

Health Policy and Disease in Colonial and Postcolonial Hong Kong, 1841–2003

Ka-che Yip, Yuen-sang Leung and
Man-kong Wong

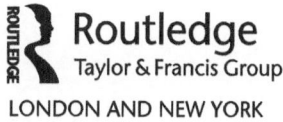

Routledge
Taylor & Francis Group

LONDON AND NEW YORK

First published 2016 by Routledge

2 Park Square, Milton Park, Abingdon, Oxfordshire OX14 4RN

711 Third Avenue, New York, NY 10017

Routledge is an imprint of the Taylor & Francis Group, an informa business

First issued in paperback 2017

British Library Cataloguing in Publication Data
A catalogue record for this book is available from the British Library

Library of Congress Cataloging-in-Publication Data
Names: Yip, Ka-che, 1944- author. | Liang, Yuansheng, author. | Huang, Wenjiang, author.
Title: Health policy and disease in colonial and Post-colonial Hong Kong, 1841-2003 / by Ka-che Yip, Philip Yuen-sang Leung, and Timothy Man-Kong Wong.
Description: Milton Park, Abingdon, Oxon ; New York, NY : Routledge, 2016. | Series: Routledge studies in the modern history of Asia ; 118 | Includes bibliographical references and index.
Identifiers: LCCN 2015049593 | ISBN 9781138943575 (hbk) | ISBN 9781315672373 (ebk)
Subjects: LCSH: Medical policy--China--Hong Kong--History. | Medical care--China--Hong Kong--History. | Epidemiology--China--Hong Kong--History.
Classification: LCC RA395.C53 Y58 2016 | DDC 362.1095125--dc23
LC record available at http://lccn.loc.gov/2015049593

ISBN: 978-1-138-94357-5 (hbk)
ISBN: 978-0-8153-5624-0 (pbk)

Typeset in Times New Roman
by Taylor & Francis Books

Contents

Acknowledgments

This study originated as a research project on the history of diseases and epidemics in Hong Kong which was supported by the Research Grant Council, Hong Kong (GRF Project Reference No. 248811). We are most grateful for the Council's financial support that made it possible for us to collect the necessary archival materials and receive the research assistance needed to complete the project. We are very much indebted to the late Dr. Lee Shiu-Hung, first director of the Hong Kong Department of Health, and subsequently professor and chair of the Department of Community and Family Medicine as well as the founding director of the School of Public Health at the Chinese University of Hong Kong, for his inspiration, encouragement, and friendship.

Throughout the preparation of this volume, we have benefitted from the research assistance of many associates, especially Dr. Law Yuen Han, whose tireless efforts are deeply appreciated. We have also received generous support from our respective home institutions: The University of Maryland Baltimore County, USA, the Chinese University of Hong Kong, and Hong Kong Baptist University. And we have received constructive criticisms from many friends and colleagues who have read sections of our work or papers presented at scholarly meetings. To all of them, our sincerest gratitude.

We would like to acknowledge the assistance of Mr. Chun-wai Li in preparing the index for this book. We also thank the Department of Health, the Government of the Hong Kong Special Administrative Region, for its permission to use the photo in the book cover.

Our special thanks to Peter Sowden at Routledge, whose interest and encouragement were invaluable throughout the process of the preparation of this book. We also thank his editorial staff for their guidance and help in the production of this volume. Finally, we are grateful to the anonymous readers who have given us useful suggestions.

1   Introduction

Objectives of the study

This book examines some of the most prevalent diseases whose historical developments were closely intertwined with the history of Hong Kong – from the establishment of the British colony in 1841 to the outbreak of the SARS epidemic in 2003, six years after it was returned to China. This time span includes the pre-World War II period of colonial rule, the Japanese occupation, the postwar era of reconstruction, the transition to decolonization from the 1980s to 1997, and the postcolonial period when Hong Kong became a Special Administrative Region (SAR) of China. This temporal coverage allows us to compare and evaluate developments in each period, from colonial to post-colonial, and during the evolution of the city from a colonial entrepot to a global financial center – an approach that will reveal the changes and continuities in disease-control policies as well as institutional adjustments and innovations.

A central concern of this study is to show how the governments – both colonial and postcolonial – dealt with the multitude of health problems associated with such diseases as malaria, smallpox, tuberculosis, plague, venereal diseases, avian influenza, and SARS (severe acute respiratory syndrome). It will illuminate how various diseases and epidemics helped to shape the emergence of strategies as well as machineries of government designed to control health problems deemed threats to the economic, social and political wellbeing of the city. The study also examines the changing perceptions of diseases among the Chinese and non-Chinese populations as well as the impact on, and responses to, diseases among different social groups and organizations. It reveals how the formulation and implementation of policies were often results of negotiation among various groups, vested interests, and the state. Finally, it looks at how Hong Kong's health status had been, and continues to be affected by the spatial spread of diseases and epidemics from other areas, especially those adjacent to the city. In short, we are interested in understanding the occurrences and consequences of diseases in the political, social, economic, and cultural context of Hong Kong history during the period under discussion. The authors have conducted research in the Hong Kong Public Records

Office, collections in the Hong Kong Museum of Medical Sciences, archives of hospitals and charitable organizations, and newspaper collections, as well as conducted oral history interviews with key individuals involved in, or knowledgeable of, the events under discussion.

Significance and contribution to scholarship

The book fills an important gap not only in the scholarship of Hong Kong studies, but also in colonial and postcolonial studies. No other studies have investigated and compared the history of diseases and epidemics over the broad sweep of time covered in this book. Studies on diseases and epidemics in Hong Kong have been either episodic narratives or records of specific diseases. With the recent outbreaks of avian influenza, SARS and other emerging diseases, scholarship has become present-minded and often treats 1997 as the "great divide" in Hong Kong history. This study is unique in its comprehensiveness and analysis, and is solidly grounded in the context of historical developments in Hong Kong. It also provides the basis for comparative studies with other colonial and postcolonial states in Asia and other parts of the world. Moreover, globalization has enhanced the potential for the outbreak of pandemics of emergent diseases or diseases previously under control, and this study will offer lessons and insights into ways to understand and combat these potential health threats.

As far as specific studies on the history of diseases in Hong Kong are concerned, David R. Phillips, in his *The Epidemiological Transition in Hong Kong: Changes in Health and Disease since the Nineteenth Century*, has investigated the changes in the disease profile in Hong Kong. The monograph is a rather technical study and does not provide the requisite historical developments of the political, economic, social, and cultural milieu within which the changes took place. A general study of the historical developments of some of the most common communicable diseases is *Plague, SARS and the Story of Medicine in Hong Kong*, although the narrative is episodic, and it also includes sections on histories of hospitals and medical education.[1] There are a number of studies on particular diseases, such as malaria, plague, venereal disease, and SARS. In his book chapter on malaria in Hong Kong history, Ka-che Yip has analyzed the complex process of policy formation on the part of the colonial government in dealing with malaria and how such policies related to public health developments in the colony.[2] Although there are articles and book chapters on plague, there are still no full-length studies. Elizabeth Sinn and Carol Benedict have examined the origin and spread of the epidemic, noting the development of government policy and local responses.[3] Except for Edward G. Pryor's article which focuses on the epidemic in Hong Kong, works by Carney T. Fisher, Myron Echenberg, and Mary P. Stuphen have tried to put Hong Kong's plague epidemic into a larger comparative context of Chinese or global history.[4] Kerrie L. MacPherson, and Phillippa Levine have written important studies on venereal diseases, examining colonial policies on prostitution, the implications of the politics on controlling bodies, and comparing attempts to combat the diseases in the British Empire.[5] SARS, not surprisingly, has received a lot of attention although many of the studies are technical in nature. Useful studies include Harris S. Ali and Roger Keil's *Networked Disease: Emerging Infections in the Global City*, Thomas Abraham's *Twenty-first Century Plague*, and Christine Loh's *At the Epicenter, Hong Kong and the SARS Outbreak*.[6] Angela Ki Che Leung and Charlotte Furth have recently edited a volume that includes studies on SARS and traditional Chinese medicine in south China, though not specifically on Hong Kong.[7]

Generally, studies on the development of health care and medical services in Hong Kong also include some discussions of various disease outbreaks. Elizabeth Sinn's study of the Tung Wah Hospital, mentioned earlier, offers an important analysis of the contributions of the Chinese local elites in providing medical services for the Chinese population. Robin Hutcheon has also examined the role of hospitals in the development of health care in Hong Kong, while Gerald H. Choa's works review the history of Hong Kong's medical services.[8] Victor C.W. Wong's study of health care development and reforms in Hong Kong offers important insights into changes in health policy and their underlying rationales.[9] Two interesting studies that compare colonial health policies in the British Empire are Margaret Jones's study of Ceylon and the Asian colonies and Law Yuen Han's study of Hong Kong and Singapore.[10]

This brief review of current scholarship reveals the lack of scholarly studies on the history of diseases and health care policies in Hong Kong that examine the changes and continuities in disease-control strategies and policies during its long history, from the colonial days to the postcolonial period. This volume therefore fills that important gap in the scholarship.

Disease control in the colonial and postcolonial state

It would be too simplistic and indeed incorrect to maintain that the British in colonial Hong Kong were merely trying to transfer hygienic or health models from their homeland when they formulated health and disease-control policies to protect themselves from the inhospitable environment and unknown diseases. Yet, they did bring with them not only contemporary ideas of health and disease, but also their cultural assumptions and perceptions of the indigenous population's way of life and backwardness, as well as their belief in the superiority of Western culture, institutions, and medical science. Social segregation of the poorer Chinese population in the Taipingshan area and the creation of enclaves for the Europeans, especially in the Peak area, was one of the ways to protect themselves from the unsanitary and unhealthy indigenous quarters. But pathogens knew no boundaries, and government intervention was necessary, especially during crises such as the plague epidemic in 1894, to ensure the social and economic wellbeing of the colony; after all, economic imperatives trumped other considerations as economic growth depended on a healthy labor force and the avoidance of being labelled an infected port.

Advances in biomedicine also provided justification for additional government attempts to regulate and "civilize" the behavior and lifestyle of the Chinese population: for example, the campaign to outlaw spitting as an anti-tuberculosis measure, or the mandatory vaccination of newborns to combat the spread of smallpox. The colonial government, however, was unwilling to invest heavily in the construction of a sanitary infrastructure, or improvements in housing, partly because of opposition from local property owners and partly because of London's reluctance to shoulder the financial burden of such projects. In the post-war period, the colonial government maintained its economics-first priority in the formulation of health policies, and as Hong Kong grew in prosperity and population, the government became more proactive in disease-control activities, and housing and environmental improvements so as to guarantee Hong Kong's sustained economic expansion. At the same time, it began to turn its attention increasingly to curative services as Hong Kong's disease-control measures had proved to be quite successful in controlling infectious diseases by the mid-1960s.

Yet, one cannot ignore local dynamics that were at work, especially the culture and social structure and beliefs of the Chinese population, the influence of the emerging Chinese elite and the entrenched power of the Europeans, and the roles played by Christian missionaries and foreign or local philanthropic organizations. The postwar period saw external forces exerting even greater impact on the making of health policies: the rise of the People's Republic of China (PRC) and the economic and political consequences for the colony that affected health policy formulation, the end of the Cold War and opening of the PRC that resulted in increased cross-border traffic between Hong Kong and China and the potential for the spread of diseases, the transition to decolonization beginning in the 1980s as Britain agreed to the return of sovereignty to the PRC in 1997; and significantly, the pandemics of newly emergent diseases and advances in biomedical science in the 1980s and 1990s.

Postcolonial Hong Kong, which became a Special Administrative Region (SAR) of the PRC, inherited the public health system and disease-control measures of its colonial past. Enjoying the freedom enshrined in the "one country, two systems" formula, Hong Kong essentially continued the economics-first priority and rejection of the welfare state principle in health policy formulation, while maintaining the basic public health infrastructure and institutions from the colonial era. Yet, local realities and developments, especially the aging population, the rise of non-communicable and chronic diseases, the legalization of traditional Chinese medicine; the growth of regional industrial and populations centers in the Pearl River Delta, as well as the threat of newly emergent diseases such as avian flu, AIDS, and SARS, and advances in biomedical research, all helped to shape health policies and disease-control approaches in postcolonial Hong Kong. Viewed from the broad perspective of Hong Kong history, we argue that the development of disease-control policies in the colonial and postcolonial periods lay at the intersections of state power, economics, culture, and science over time as well as at specific situations, all of them interacting in a local, regional, and international milieu.

Summary of chapters

Following a brief discussion in the Introduction of the objectives and significance of this study and how it fits into the existing body of scholarship, Chapter 2 explores the dynamics of colonial health policy formation, focusing especially on the cultural, social, and economic dimensions of disease control during the early decades of colonial rule when the government was adjusting to changing conditions in the colony. It examines if there were direct policy transfers from the metropolitan center to the colony and how, if any, were they modified to meet local realities. The chapter reveals that health and disease-control policies often resulted from complex processes of negotiations among different groups and vested interests. The British had to devise strategies to deal with an unfamiliar environment and unknown diseases, the most prevalent of which included malaria, cholera, typhoid, smallpox, measles, tuberculosis, and venereal diseases. These diseases constituted one of the most serious threats to the health of the colonials, not to mention the economic viability of the colony. The increase in population – partly a result of the periodic influx of migrants from China who might help to spread pathogens – and the lack of housing for the poor, led to overcrowding and created ideal conditions for the spread of communicable diseases. The government tended to adopt a relatively hands-free attitude in health matters toward the Chinese population, most of whom utilized traditional Chinese medicine, as long as there were no serious outbreaks that would threaten the social and economic wellbeing of the colony, although Europeans generally attributed the causes of many of the diseases to the unsanitary conditions in the Chinese community. Segregation measures barring Chinese from specific areas were introduced and voluntary and charitable organizations provided some relief for those Chinese seeking help. Instead of long-term planning for the building of an adequate sanitary infrastructure as recommended by expert studies, the government only introduced environmental improvements and sanitary reforms piecemeal. The outbreak of the plague epidemic in 1894 in the Chinese community of Taipingshan marked a turning point in the evolution of health policies in the colony. The government, reacting to the severity of the situation, especially the threat to the economy, imposed political, social, and cultural sanctions, including the use of troops to dislodge families and forcibly remove patients; it also assumed the supervision of Tung Wah Hospital which had serviced the Chinese population with traditional Chinese medicine.

Chapter 3 studies the aftermath and consequences of the plague epidemic. Increased government intervention coincided to some extent with advances in scientific medicine. For example, the discovery of the plague bacilli led to the implementation of measures to reduce the rodent population and mandatory house cleaning. With the identification of the anopheles as the carrier of malaria parasites, the government began scientific investigation of malaria including the collection of mosquito specimens and strengthened its anti-vector measures focusing on the construction of drains and sewers. Vaccination against smallpox became law, and variolation, commonly used by the Chinese, was banned. A major concern of this chapter is to examine how current medical knowledge, cultural and racial assumptions, as well as local social and economic imperatives shaped health and disease-control policies at that time. It shows that many Chinese were not passive recipients of modern medical science, and they often reacted with skepticism and even resistance. At the same time, it examines how medical emergencies and the authority of biomedicine contributed to the emergence of institutions and routinization of practices that strengthened the state's control while enhancing the wellbeing and stability of the city that were deemed vital to its economic growth.

Chapter 4 looks at how population growth, changing demographics, urbanization, and the evolving economy contributed to changing morbidity and mortality rates and changes in government attempts to control disease outbreaks during the interwar years. By the 1930s, the continued urbanization, environmental improvements, and better drainage of the island resulted in a steady decline in malaria infection in Hong Kong and Kowloon although many cases persisted in the New Territories. Smallpox mortality also began to decline. Yet the government's failure to address the problem of unsanitary and congested housing meant that tuberculosis and other diseases such as enteritis remained serious threats in the early twentieth century, especially with the rapid industrialization of the city in the interwar years when many small apartments became workshops with deplorable hygienic conditions. This chapter studies how the government reconciled the desire to economize and the need to expend resources to maintain a healthy environment for workers and a disease-free port. It explains how local economic and social imperatives shaped health and disease-control policies during this period of rapid industrialization, changing demographics, as well as overcrowding and poverty for large segments of the growing population. The Japanese invasion in December 1941 and subsequent occupation of Hong Kong resulted in serious damages to the health infrastructure and services, including supplies of medicines and food. There was a resurgence of malaria, and a rise in the morbidity rate of tuberculosis, venereal disease, beriberi, and deficiency diseases.

During the early postwar period, Hong Kong expended much effort on political and economic reconstruction, and Chapter 5 concerns the factors shaping the formation of health policies and disease-control measures, and their implementation. Anxious to rebuild a public health infrastructure to ensure a healthy labor force and a disease-free port, the government, while still adopting a tight fiscal policy, concentrated its health resources on public health improvements in general and anti-disease activities in particular through the mid-1960s. Factors such as the tremendous influx of mainland refugees after 1949, many of whom had to live in squatters because of the lack of housing, as well as the rising dissatisfaction with social inequality and poor living and working conditions were important factors that prompted the government to begin public housing planning and construction as well as the development of new towns in the New Territories. Moreover, it focused on the control and prevention of communicable diseases, immunization campaigns, health education, free health care for patients of most infectious diseases, and the development of maternal and child care services. The chapter argues that while the government was not interested in the creation of a welfare state, it did recognize the need to alleviate social tension through the provision of basic public health services – which would further develop a healthy environment for Hong Kong's economic transformation and expansion – even when relatively little was done to expand curative services for the population.

Chapter 6 focuses on the epidemiological transition after the mid-1960s and the government's shift to emphasizing more on curative services as Hong Kong's disease profile had changed from one dominated by infectious diseases to one characterized by heart diseases, cancer, and other diseases associated with aging – characteristics of the disease profile of a modern "developed" society. The transition resulted from the success of anti-communicable disease measures, changing demographics, improvements in living standards, the continued urbanization of the city, and the rising life expectancy. The chapter also examines the social and political dynamics that helped to shape the government's health polices: the social unrest of the 1960s, the need to enhance the prestige of the government and ease social tension, and the unprecedented economic prosperity which allowed an expansion of programs in housing, education, social welfare, and medical services. The specter of epidemics remained, however, as urbanization and globalization facilitated the spread of emerging infectious diseases caused by new strains of viruses or newly discovered viruses. The pandemic of the "Hong Kong flu" of 1968 and the emergence of HIV/AIDS in the early 1980s led to a greater emphasis on a system of disease surveillance as Hong Kong, now a world city and financial hub, tried to be vigilant in protecting the city and its people from imported diseases.

With the Joint Declaration of December 1984 which set July 1, 1997 as the date of the return of Hong Kong to China, Hong Kong's de facto decolonization began. Chapter 7 examines how the prolonged transition to 1997 impacted the colony's health and disease-control polices during a period of uncertainty. To inspire confidence, the government continued to proclaim its intention to safeguard and promote the general public health of the community through investment in public health, especially when there was a resurgence of some communicable diseases resulting from the influx of Vietnamese refugees. It also stressed the provision of health services to the needy. A second medical school was opened to train more doctors for the growing, more affluent, and aging, population. An attempt to provide more equitable health care to different regions led to the adoption of a regionalization of public care at the local level. The government also separated the management of public health, including disease control and prevention, and medical care functions; the former would reside with the Health Department, while the latter would be under the control of a newly created Hospital Authority. The chapter argues that with the impending retrocession of Hong Kong, the government was making incremental changes to accommodate the realities of the new socio-economic conditions with priority given to maintaining a healthy environment but was reluctant to make fundamental changes to the system and putatively sensitive decisions were postponed.

The major concerns of Chapter 8 are first, to examine the public health system and disease-control measures in a postcolonial state; and second, to study how the government dealt with the outbreaks of major pandemics – from avian flu to SARS – and evaluate the strengths and weaknesses of the city's disease prevention and surveillance systems. Were there major changes and innovations – institutional as well as approaches – after 1997? What was the legacy of the colonial period? The government also had to devise new strategies to deal with health problems associated with the growing aging population, the rise of chronic diseases, and the impact of environmental problems. Moreover, closer ties with China and the surge in cross-border traffic also brought new challenges to disease prevention and control. Hong Kong has been in the forefront of scientific investigations into the avian flu and SARS: in fact, Hong Kong scientists first described the coronavirus that caused SARS in 2003. Hong Kong cooperated closely with WHO and other international agencies to monitor and control the spread of the pandemic. This chapter studies Hong Kong's handling of the SARS crisis and its role in combating emergent global diseases. It evaluates how its health and research infrastructure which has been developing over time – from the colonial to the postcolonial period – helps to protect Hong Kong from future disease outbreaks.

Notes

1 David R. Phillips, *The Epidemiological Transition in Hong Kong: Changes in Health and Disease since the Nineteenth Century* (Hong Kong: Center of Asian Studies, University of Hong Kong, 1988); Arthur Starling et al., *Plague, SARS and the Story of Medicine in Hong Kong* (Hong Kong: Hong Kong University Press, 2006).
2 Ka-che Yip, "Colonialism, Disease, and Public Health: Malaria in the History of Hong Kong," in Ka-che Yip ed., *Disease, Colonialism, and the State: Malaria in Modern East Asian History* (Hong Kong: Hong Kong University Press, 2009), 11–30.
3 Elizabeth Sinn, *Power and Charity: The Early History of the Tung Wah Hospital* (Hong Kong: Oxford University Press, 1989); and Carol Benedict, *Bubonic Plague in Nineteenth-Century China* (Stanford: Stanford University Press, 1996).
4 Edward G. Pryor, "The Great Plague of Hong Kong," *Journal of the Hong Kong Branch of the Royal Asiatic Society*, 15 (1975), 61–70; Carney T. Fisher, "The Plague in Chinese History," in Mark Elvin and Liu Ts'ui-jung eds., *Sediments of Time: Environment and Society in Chinese History* (Taipei: Academia Sinica, 1995), 673–745; Myron Echenberg, *Plague Ports: the Global Urban Impact of Bubonic Plague, 1894–1901* (New York: New York University Press, 2007); Mary P. Sutphen, "Not What, But Where: Bubonic Plague and the Reception of Germ Theories in Hong Kong and Calcutta, 1894–1897," *Journal of the History of*

Medicine and Allied Sciences, 52:1 (1997), 81–113; and her "Rumoured Power: Hong Kong, 1894 and Cape Town, 1901," in Andrew Cunningham and Bridie Andrews eds., *Western Medicine as Contested Knowledge* (Manchester: Manchester University Press, 1997), 241–261.

5 Phillippa Levine, *Prostitution, Race, and Politics: Policing Venereal Disease in the British Empire* (New York: Routledge, 2003), and her "Modernity, Medicine and Colonialism: The Contagious Diseases Ordinances in Hong Kong and the Straits Settlements," *Positions*, 6:3 (1998), 675–705; Kerrie L. MacPherson, "Health and Empire: Britain's National Campaign to Combat Venereal Diseases in Shanghai, Hong Kong and Singapore," in R. Davidson et al., *Sex, Sin and Suffering: Venereal Disease and European Society since 1870* (London: Routledge, 2001), 173–190.

6 Harris S. Ali and Roger Keil eds., *Networked Disease: Emerging Infections in the Global City* (Chichester, UK: Wiley-Blackwell, 2008); Thomas Abraham, *Twenty-first Century Plague: The Story of SARS* (Hong Kong: Hong Kong University Press, 2004); Christine Loh et al., *At the Epicenter: Hong Kong and the SARS Outbreak* (Hong Kong: Hong Kong University Press), 2004.

7 Angela Ki Che Leung and Charlotte Furth eds., *Health and Hygiene in Chinese East Asia: Policies and Publics in the Long Twentieth Century* (Durham: Duke University Press, 2011).

8 Robin Hutcheon, *Bedside Manner: Hospital and Health Care in Hong Kong* (Hong Kong: The Chinese University Press, 1999); Gerald H. Choa, "A History of Medicine in Hong Kong," in *Medical Directory of Hong Kong* (Hong Kong: The Federation of Medical Societies of Hong Kong, 1985), 13–29; and his "Hong Kong's Health and Medical Services," in Albert H. Yee ed., *Whither Hong Kong: China's Shadow or Visionary Gleam* (Lanham: University Press of America, 1999), 153–186.

9 Victor C. W. Wong, *The Political Economy of Health Care Development and Reform in Hong Kong* (Aldershop: Ashgate, 1999).

10 Margaret Jones, "British Colonial Health Policy, 1900–1949: Ceylon and the Asian Colonies," Ph.D. thesis, University of Bristol, 2000; Luo Wanxian [Law Yuen Han], "Xifang yixue yu zhimin guanzhi: yi erci shijie dazhan qian Xianggang he Xinjiapo wei bijiao gean" [Western Medicine and Colonial Rule: Pre-WWII Hong Kong and Singapore as Comparative Cases], Ph.D. thesis, Hong Kong Baptist University, 2007.

2   Disease-control policies, 1841–1894
Colonial priorities and local realities

The inception of colonial rule and its policy priorities

Hong Kong was occupied by the British in late January 1841, and although the British Foreign Secretary Lord Palmerston dismissed it as a "barren rock,"[1] Britain decided to include China's cession of Hong Kong as one of the terms of the Nanjing Treaty that concluded the Opium War in 1842. The British government and the British mercantile community were interested in developing free trade in the colony; in January 1843, the new Foreign Secretary Lord Aberdeen directed Henry Pottinger, the colony's first governor, to turn Hong Kong into a "great mercantile entrepot where the harbor dues should... be as light as possible, so as to give every encouragement to the commerce of all nations."[2] The hope, however, was not realized, at least in the first decade of British rule as China trade failed to develop, and businesses and even the Hong Kong government suffered loss and budget deficits.

For the British colonials, the hot and humid climate and the inland marshes and swamps had led them to believe that Hong Kong was an unhealthy place when the colony was first established. The most prevalent diseases in the colony included malaria, cholera, tuberculosis, smallpox, and dysentery. Although a rudimentary medical service was established with the appointment of a Colonial Surgeon in 1843,[3] not much was done to improve the topographical environment or sanitary infrastructure. An anonymous letter published in *The Friends of China*, pointed out that the hope of Hong Kong developing into an entrepot for trade with China would be dashed because of "the general sickness that prevails."[4] The view that Hong Kong's disease problems would negatively impact its future was shared by Robert M. Martin, the colonial treasurer. Martin, trained as a surgeon, cited disease as a major factor inhibiting Hong Kong's future development. In particular, he pointed to the numerous health problems confronting the troops in the colony. According to him, in 1845 alone, every man from the European and native troops had visited the hospital more than five times! Fever, diarrhea, and dysentery were prevalent; and in addition to deaths, many men became unfit for duty as a result of illness. Martin subscribed to the contemporary belief that diseases resulted from "destructive miasma" caused by heavy rainfall and inadequate drainage, conditions that helped to generate "noxious vapor rising from putrescent organic matter, marshland, etc. which polluted the atmosphere" and caused illness.[5]

However, a select committee dispatched by London in 1847 to investigate trading conditions in Hong Kong concluded that the colony had significant potential for China trade.[6] Political and social unrest in China, especially during the Taiping Rebellion that broke out in 1850, resulted in the relocation of some well-off Chinese to Hong Kong. Their presence and financial connections in China contributed to the colony's growing prosperity. In 1860, as a result of China's defeat in the Second Opium War, Britain added the Kowloon Peninsula to the colony. The ensuing decades saw further growth of the port of Hong Kong in the China trade, and by the mid-1890s, Hong Kong emerged as the entrepot for nearly half of China's foreign trade.[7] A Convention between China and Britain in 1898 further expanded Hong Kong's territory to the boundary with China, adding the leased New Territories in the process, and assuring Britain firm control of the excellent Victoria Harbor. By the turn of the century, Hong Kong had become a prosperous city with a growing population – 7,450 in 1841 and over 300,000 in 1898.[8]

Throughout this period, the government maintained a laissez-faire policy toward trade; it also refrained from making any substantial investment in infrastructural improvements for the colony. In spite of the growing population, there was no policy in housing and welfare; only a minimal investment from the government, however, was put in public education.[9] This was a sentiment shared by the mercantile community, European and Asian alike, who, while trying to maximize profits, were also only making the minimum requisite investment in the construction of piers and warehouses. This, however, did not prevent Hong Kong from emerging into a hub of entrepot trade as it was able to tap into the multi-layered networks of China trade within the trading system of treaty ports in coastal China and Southeast Asian ports.

A minimal interventionist approach also underlay the government's social and health policies in general, especially toward the Chinese population. In spite of the growing population, most of them Chinese, the government had no long-term housing or welfare policies. Local voluntarism, including initiatives from foreign missionaries and affluent members of the mercantile community, sometimes helped to compensate for the government's lack of initiatives. The government likewise adopted a relatively hands-free attitude as far as health matters were concerned; and its econometric approach to health dictated that under the tight budget policy, outlays on public health improvements would be minimal, but hopefully adequate to maintain a healthy labor force to ensure economic growth. Disease-control measures therefore tended to be piecemeal and ad hoc. Yet when there were disease outbreaks that would pose a serious threat to the public in general and members of the British community in particular, the government would intervene quickly, and even forcibly, to protect what it viewed as the social and economic wellbeing of the colony.

Racial attitudes and disease control

A major issue that the colonial government had to deal with was the influx of Chinese migrants during this period, especially in the 1850s when the Taiping Rebellion caused much social upheaval in China, and the 1880s and 1890s when the burgeoning economy of Hong Kong attracted a large number of newcomers seeking jobs. Without any clearly defined urban planning policy, the British encouraged the poor migrants to settle in the Taipingshan area; in fact, in 1844, Chinese newcomers were forced to relocate there.[10] The surge in the Chinese population during this period: from 31,463 in 1851 to 61,952 in 1861, and from 96,856 in 1881 to 136,901 in 1891, resulted in the concentration of a large number of residents in a small urban ghetto with poor housing and deplorable sanitary conditions that would be a hotbed for diseases.[11] The 1850s indeed saw sporadic disease outbreaks among the Chinese community. For example, between February 6 and April 28, 1856, of the 799 deaths among the Chinese population caused by fever and other acute diseases, 379 were from the Taipingshan area. C. May, the Registrar-General, refused to acknowledge the severity of the problem; he simply claimed that as far as incidences of diseases were concerned, "[t]he district of Taipingshan has a small excess over the other districts."[12]

Yet, racial attitudes and colonial mentality among the British buttressed their belief that the Chinese population was in fact part of the health problems in the colony. The prevalence of diseases was linked to the "filthy habits of life amongst the…Chinese," and the cultural practices and overcrowded and unsanitary living conditions of the Chinese were threats to the Western civilized way of life.[13] In India, the British had established "hill stations" where they could escape from the heat and humidity and the undesirable lifestyle of the indigenous population. In Hong Kong, the British were ready to concede that "unlike the Chinese who have probably by a long process of natural selection, become inured and insensible to the conditions inseparable from extreme density of population, they are rendered ill and miserable by the effects of habits which such insensibility produces."[14]

To protect themselves and to control the spread of disease, the government moved to reserve certain areas in the colony for only European-style housing. The European District Reservation Ordinance that became effective on February 20, 1889 disallowed any building of Chinese tenements as well as sub-divisions of any room or floor less than 1,000 cubic feet in parts of present-day Midlevel and the Peak areas. The Chinese could still own buildings that conformed to the European building requirements in the district.[15] But after the plague epidemic of 1894, a more restrictive ordinance was passed in 1904 that reserved the Peak area for Westerners only, excluding Chinese and even Eurasians from that area.[16] The military, always concerned with the wellbeing of the troops, reacted to a report in 1874 by the Colonial Surgeon that painted a grim picture of the unhygienic living conditions in the Chinese tenements by insisting that no such housing should be allowed in the neighborhoods of barracks. The Governor assured the military that "the new buildings near the barracks were built to higher-than-usual standards."[17]

Housing, sanitary reforms, and disease control

Social segregation, however, could not stop the spread of pathogens. The segregationist policy assumed that as long as the Chinese lived apart and that no major health problems arose, there was no need to pay much attention to the conditions of the Chinese population. The poor living conditions in the overcrowded Chinese tenements did attract the attention of colonial officials who warned about the potential health hazards in the Taipingshan area. Nothing substantial was done, however, to improve the general problems of sanitation, partly because of opposition from property owners, and partly because London wanted assurance that local funds were available for such projects.[18] In 1881, London invited Osbert Chadwick to investigate the situation in the colony. Osbert Chadwick's father, Edwin Chadwick, was a pioneer in sanitation reforms and his investigation into the sanitary conditions of the working class made possible the passage of the first public health legislation in Britain in 1848.[19] A professional engineer by training, Osbert Chadwick promoted public health reforms through better architectural and engineering designs. His investigation covered the entire City of Victoria while paying special attention to the conditions of tenements occupied by the Chinese. He noted that congested conditions existed outside the Taipingshan area as well, and the most common practice contributing to congestion was that flats were often sub-divided into smaller units. This practice caused unhealthy and deplorable living conditions especially among the poor. He wrote:

> The lodging houses of common labourers are often very much crowded. In a row of eight small houses 428 inhabitants were found, having but 230 cubic feet of space per head, exclusive of the cookhouse. These houses were exceedingly filthy. They were built close to the scrap of the hill, from which they were separated by a narrow gully only, which was wet and very dirty, and without proper drainage.[20]

Chadwick's report, released a year later, recommended improvements in drainage and sewage, water supply, and upgrades in the building code that would require more open spaces. The Hong Kong government appointed a sanitary inspector in 1883 to oversee the new Sanitary Section within the Survey Department, and a Sanitary Board was also established to advise the government on changes in building requirements. It, however, was not prepared to invest heavily in the construction of a better sanitary infrastructure. Instead, its priority was to improve the filthy conditions and remove the sources of noxious odour or miasma through better ventilation within and between buildings. In 1886, Acting Governor Henry Marsh initiated the drafting of a Public Health Ordinance that would mandate the inclusion of space within and without the buildings, including backyard space and the space between buildings.[21]

The draft bill received a cool reception when it was discussed in the Sanitary Board in December 1886, partly because of the presence of Dr. Ho Kai, a practitioner of Western medicine and a practicing lawyer in Hong Kong,[22] and Dr. Patrick Manson, already well-known for his medical research in China and Britain. Medical practitioners in Britain and Hong Kong did not take the Chakwicks seriously, as both father and son had not studied medicine which, in the view of its practitioners, was far superior to engineering in solving what were perceived to be medical problems. Ho, a well-respected member of Hong Kong society, was adamant that the Chinese did not require housing improvements imposed on them by Europeans. Moreover, since there was a constant influx of people from south China providing a cheap source of labor, the demand for inexpensive temporary housing would remain strong. The ordinance, he argued, would in fact force the poor to live in even smaller spaces, and would not achieve its objective of improving the general sanitary conditions.[23] The government did not want to undermine the consultative relationship with the Sanitary Board that it hoped would lead to a more effective governance system through consensus building with Chinese social leaders whom they empowered and trusted.[24] This approach applied to public health as well as other issues.

Controlling infectious diseases

The most prevalent infectious diseases during this period included malaria, tuberculosis, smallpox, cholera, and venereal diseases. The term "Hong Kong fever" was commonly used to describe various types of fever, but by the 1890s, it was determined that "Hong Kong fever" was, in most cases, malaria. Hong Kong's topography, and hot humid climate proved to be ideal for the breeding of mosquitoes, although it was not until the end of the nineteenth century that mosquitoes were shown to be a vector of the disease. An outbreak of Hong Kong fever was recorded in June 1841; and between May and October 1843, "24% of troops and 10% of European civilians died of fever."[25] At that time, malaria was viewed as an environmental problem and malarial miasma resulted from decomposing vegetation in marshes and swamps. Before 1890, the Colonial Surgeon's annual reports did not list malaria separately, and it is difficult to have exact figures of malaria morbidity.[26] Tuberculosis, or phthisis, was also viewed as associated with filth and impure air, and from the mid-nineteenth century, open air and rest therapies became popular throughout Europe and the United States as the remedy for tuberculosis patients. Not surprisingly, the poor living conditions of the Chinese were viewed with dismay by Europeans as providing the ideal environment for tuberculosis and other diseases. Reports of the Colonial Surgeon did not contain much specific information on the diseases, and there was no specific section on tuberculosis. The 1877 report, for example, noted that there were 14 phthisis admissions to the Civil Hospital and half of those patients died.[27] Tuberculosis was not one of the pressing health issues, it was chronic in nature and did not create the dramatic sense of urgency as plague or other epidemics.

Early statistics also did not reveal the true dimension of the problem of smallpox which was endemic in Hong Kong, although colonial medical officials had noted the "very excessive" smallpox mortality among the Chinese by the early 1850s.[28] To combat the spread of smallpox, Dr. J. Carroll Dempster, the Colonial Surgeon, proposed mandatory vaccination of the population. At that time, the government rejected the idea since there was no immediate health crisis; after all, such diseases as malaria and tuberculosis killed more people than smallpox. Anti-smallpox strategy therefore centered on the protection of individuals and communities from infection by isolation of patients, and the government would not intervene as long as there were no widespread outbreaks. There were however small smallpox epidemics, for example in 1887–1888 when 374 died.[29] Finally, in 1890, the government passed a Vaccination Ordinance mandating the vaccination of infants within six months after birth. The Ordinance was difficult to enforce since the tracking of infants arriving or being taken to China by their parents remained problematic.[30] But by the 1890s, the number of Chinese being vaccinated steadily increased, especially when the Tung Wah Hospital, which was trusted by the Chinese community, provided free vaccination service.

Unlike tuberculosis or smallpox, the control of cholera was to a significant extent affected by international developments. Hong Kong was affected by the third pandemic of cholera (1852–1859) when the first authenticated case of cholera was identified in 1858, although there were no exact figures of case mortality. Hong Kong did not experience major cholera outbreaks until the early twentieth century. But cholera was a disease subject to international quarantine, and Hong Kong, as an international port, was of course cautious about cholera outbreaks elsewhere. In 1883, many ships were in quarantine in Hong Kong harbor when cholera outbreaks occurred in southeastern China and the Philippines. There had been attempts among the international community to establish guidelines to control the spread of the disease; Britain, concerned with the economic impact of quarantine on maritime trade, had insisted that domestic sanitary and public health reforms were more useful. Hong Kong already had a quarantine system in place since many ports required Bills of Health for ships coming from Hong Kong. In 1884, when the Governor requested clarifications from London regarding quarantine, he was told that Hong Kong should maintain its system since unsanitary conditions in the colony were conducive to the spread of diseases if there were no quarantine control.[31]

The troops stationed in Hong Kong were of course very much affected by the prevalence of infectious diseases. The military, in fact, had been keeping close tabs on the health conditions of the military personnel. Health reports of the troops in Hong Kong, including the number of soldiers who had died or were stricken with diseases were presented to the War Office in London at regular intervals. One specific concern was the spread of venereal diseases among the troops. The Contagious Disease Act, passed in November 1857, mandated the registration of brothels. Moreover, prostitutes were required to attend medical inspection at frequent intervals, and, if found to be infected by a venereal disease, would be removed from registered brothels and sent to the Lock Hospital, opened in 1858, for treatment. Punishments were imposed if venereal disease was transmitted by the prostitutes.[32] In fact, similar legislations were enacted in other parts of the British Empire where prostitutes, native or foreign, were required to go through body checks to qualify for their registration.[33] Expenses associated with the legislation were to be covered by the registration fees as well as fines from sly brothels, unregistered prostitutes, or those prostitutes who infected their customers with venereal diseases. The decline in the number of infections among troops stationed in Hong Kong in subsequent years suggested that the legislation was effective in checking the spread of venereal diseases. Yet in ensuing decades, there was growing criticism of the legislation among both the Chinese and Western communities in Hong Kong.

In the late 1870s, an accidental fall involving a prostitute led to debates over whether reforms of the Act were necessary, especially in its enforcement and the excessive power given to the inspector of brothels – even when it was for the sake of such common good as public health. Governor Hennessey appointed a committee to look into the issue. The committee split 2–1 in its recommendations, issued in late 1878 and early 1879 respectively. The majority recognized the need to respect the views and sentiments of the Chinese, especially with regard to the medical examination, and recommended that "the licenses to be granted in future should be strictly limited to houses for the accommodation of foreigners.[34] In the end, the Colonial Office decided that exemption "from all liability to medical inspection" applied to Chinese prostitutes and brothels "used by Chinese only," while surveillance of those brothels used by non-Chinese, mostly troops stationed in Hong Kong, would continue.[35] In 1886, widespread criticism of the Contagious Disease Act in Britain and across the British Empire led to its abolition by the Parliament. Forced to comply with instructions from London, the Hong Kong government resorted to the use of the Protection of Women and Girls Ordinance designed to ensure only willing women served as prostitutes to control the spread of venereal diseases through the registration of brothels. As an incentive, any infected women would receive free treatment, lodging, and meals in the hospital. Yet, venereal diseases remained a core concern for the military in Hong Kong.

Hospital services

The first decades of colonial rule set the priorities for public health and disease-control policies: a tight budget policy that reinforced the unwillingness to invest heavily in improvements of the under-developed sanitary infrastructure;

concern for the health of the European residents and troops stationed in Hong Kong; scant attention to the health and sanitary conditions of the Chinese community; and a general non-interventionist approach as long as there were no serious epidemics that threatened economic growth and social stability. The government generally adhered to these priorities even with the surge in Chinese population and the growth in China trade: between 1887 and 1896, Hong Kong accounted for 45 to 48 percent of China's total foreign trade. As early as the 1840s, Governor John F. Davis, being unable because of budget deficit, and reluctant to invest in infrastructural developments, nonetheless recognized the value of providing some sort of medical services. He subsequently oversaw the building of a government Civil Hospital that was completed in 1849. The hospital, however, did not provide medical services to the local population; it served only the police force, civil servants, convicts, the destitute, or those able to pay for the service.[36] For the wealthy, they would consult established private practitioners of Western medicine. Davis also approved a land lease for the building of a medical school proposed by Dr. Benjamin Hobson, a medical missionary who was in charge of a successful mission hospital that had attracted a large number of Chinese patrons. Unfortunately, Hobson failed to raise enough funds for the proposed school and the plan was shelved.[37]

Some Chinese traders in Hong Kong had benefited from the burgeoning China trade, and the personal wealth of some of these merchants was reflected in the fact that in 1876, eight out of the top 20 rate-payers in Hong Kong were Chinese.[38] The emergence of a wealthy Chinese elite at this time proved to be fortuitous as they were becoming more actively involved in public affairs in early Hong Kong, and would indeed play a pivotal role in addressing some of the health issues of the local Chinese population in the 1870s. The origin of the Tung Wah Hospital can be traced to the Man Mo temple, established in 1847. The temple soon became a social center for the Chinese community, and the committee overseeing the temple began to play a significant role in handling grievances and problems among the Chinese. To solve the problem of honoring properly the deceased whose bodies were not returned to their homeland – a custom to which the Chinese attached great importance – the Kwong Fuk I-tze was built for people to pay respect to ancestral tablets housed in the hall. In 1866, the Colonial Surgeon and the Inspector of Nuisance expressed concern that it had become the home for destitutes who could not afford to go to the Civil Hospital for treatment, and that conditions in the hall were poor and unhygienic. However, the government's non-interventionist approach still prevailed until 1869 when a migrant worker died in the hall. This provoked widespread concern not only in Hong Kong but also in London. Local Chinese leaders proposed to Governor Richard MacDonnell the building of a hospital for the Chinese. The construction funds were raised by the Chinese leaders, with a government subsidy of HK$115,000, an unprecedented amount spent by the government for Chinese affairs in the early history of Hong Kong. The hospital opened in 1872 for the Chinese population, and only used traditional Chinese medicine for treatment.[39] It, however, provided smallpox vaccination free of charge. As will be discussed later, the hospital would encounter much opposition from Western medical practitioners, especially during the plague epidemic of 1894.

The plague epidemic

The bubonic plague epidemic that broke out in May 1894 had far-reaching implications for subsequent developments in Hong Kong's health and disease-control policies, as well as in relations between the Chinese population and the colonial government. The plague was caused by a bacillus that was carried by fleas found in infected rats, and the disease was transmitted to humans through the bite of the fleas. The plague originated in Yunnan province in China in the 1850s and slowly spread eastward to Guangzhou, Hong Kong, and subsequently to the rest of the world in what became known as the Third Plague Pandemic. Thanks to the record left by Dr. James Lowson who was acting superintendent of the Civil Hospital at that time, we have a much fuller account of what happened in Hong Kong during the epidemic.[40]

On May 10, Hong Kong was declared an infected port. On that same day, the government decided to adopt the policy of isolation to control the spread of the disease. *Hygeia*, a medical ship that had been used to isolate patients suffering from smallpox and cholera, was pressed into service for plague patients.[41] Troops were deployed to search for infected patients who would be removed forcibly from their homes and their belongings disinfected. As panic spread through the city, many began to leave Hong Kong. The house-to-house inspections and compulsory removal of the sick in Taipingshan, the center of the epidemic, provoked unprecedented opposition from Chinese residents who objected to what they perceived as intrusiveness and insensitivities to Chinese social and cultural norms, especially when women were required to stand in public while disinfection of houses were being carried out. When the Chinese requested the cessation of house-to-house search, the removal of patients to Tung Wah Hospital, and the permission to ship the deceased to their native places for burial, the government labeled the petition "unreasonable," and even ordered the gunboat *Tweed* to station nearby with its guns pointing to Tung Wah Hospital! Amid the mounting crisis and sense of urgency, the government finally agreed to some concessions: Tung Wah Hospital would take over the management of the isolation wards at the old glass work factory in Kennedy Town that had been used for isolating patients, and the sick and bodies of the deceased were allowed to be returned to their native places. The death toll from the disease was high: in 1894 alone, out of the 2,679 cases reported, 2,485 died. While nearly 98 percent of those infected were Chinese, only 11 Europeans succumbed to the disease.[42]

The plague epidemic in Hong Kong provided the backdrop for one of the most important breakthroughs in medical science. Two bacteriologists, Dr. Shibasaburo Kitasato from Japan and Dr. Alexandre Yersin from France were in Hong Kong in June researching the plague. Although Dr. Kitasato discovered his plague bacillus nine days before Dr. Yersin discovered his, the credit of discovery went to Yersin as Kitasato's findings lacked precision and report of his findings by Dr. Lowson proved to be premature. Dr. Tom Solomon who had studied the controversy, pointed to Dr. Lowson's rush to publish the results as partly responsible for costing Kitasato his claim to the credit.[43] Although the bacillus was identified, yet the riddle was only half-solved. It was not until a decade later that the Indian Plague Investigation Committee was able to identify fleas as agents for the transmission of bacillus between rats and humans. An effective cure was only available in 1938, while a more highly effective one came into use in 1946. Between 1895 and 1929, plague returned to Hong Kong every year, "beginning in February or March, peaking in June, and fading away in the early autumn."[44]

By October 1894, the situation in Hong Kong improved and the number of cases decreased. In September 1894, the government passed an ordinance of resumption of properties in Taipingshan and demolished buildings that were deemed necessary to prevent a recurrence of plague. A sizable piece of land was turned into a public garden – the Blake Garden. Some new houses were built according to upgraded sanitary codes and new requirements of space usage.[45] Other parts of the city also received regular cleaning to rid the filth and pest population that might create conditions for disease outbreaks. The government also introduced a nascent form of rat-control policy. At first, financial incentives were given according to the numbers of rats caught, but the practice was soon discontinued because people began to import rats from South China.[46] At the same time, Dr. Lowson, in his report on the epidemic, demanded that Western medicine should be introduced and used in the Tung Wah Hospital, a position originally advocated by the then acting Colonial Surgeon in 1872. The government indeed extended its control and supervision over the hospital, and a Chinese practitioner of Western medicine, Dr. Chung King U, left his position in the Alice Memorial Hospital for Tung Wah, which, however, was allowed to continue using Chinese medical treatment as well.[47]

The plague epidemic revealed clearly the government's priorities in disease control. As an infected port, Hong Kong suffered tremendous economic loss as ships shunned the colony, thereby jeopardizing the colony's premier position in international trade. The exodus of people from Hong Kong crippled manufacturing and building projects. Prices in the colony began to rise, and as panic mounted, there seemed to be a genuine threat to public order.[48] From the government's point of view, social wellbeing and economic viability of the colony were at stake. The hitherto laissez faire policy had to be modified to deal with the urgent threat. It therefore had to intervene quickly and forcibly, even though it meant the implementation of intrusive measures and risked confrontation with the Chinese community. The plague epidemic also helped to reinforce the dominant position of Western biomedicine in Hong Kong. Although traditional Chinese medicine was tolerated by the government and was used by the overwhelmingly majority of the Chinese population for medical relief, it was marginalized and would never receive official recognition and be incorporated into the colony's health care system. New ordinances to improve sanitary conditions, housing, and the use of urban space would follow. As an international port, the plague epidemic, as in the case of cholera, revealed clearly how both domestic and international factors affected Hong Kong's attempt to control diseases. The Kitasato–Yersin efforts at the end of the century marked a new page in medical research which was gaining increasing prominence in shaping disease-control policies and strategies – a theme that will be discussed in detail in the next chapter.

Notes

1 Susanna Hoe and Derek Roebuck, *The Taking of Hong Kong: Charles and Clara Elliot in China Waters* (London: Curzon, 1999), 156–159.
2 "Lord Aberdeen to Governor Henry Pottinger, 4 January 1843," cited in Steve Tsang, *A Documentary History of Hong Kong: Government and Politics* (Hong Kong: Hong Kong University Press, 1995), 17.
3 The post was named Colonial Surgeon although there was no colonial hospital. His two consecutive successors also left the post after a brief period of service, resigning because of personal health reasons. It was only after the establishment of the Civil Hospital that the colonial surgeons played a clearer and more defined role. See Ho Pui Yin, *The Administrative History of the Government Agencies, 1841–2002* (Hong Kong: Hong Kong University Press, 2004).
4 "Original Correspondence (25 September 1843)," *The Friends of China and Hong Kong Gazette* (October 5, 1843).
5 R. M. Martin, "Report on Hong Kong in all its aspects (August 1844)," in *Reports, Minutes and Dispatches on the British Position and Prospects in China* (London: Harrison and Co. Printers, 1846), 7–12. It should be noted that his report was circulated and read at the British Parliament. See *British Parliamentary Papers: China.* Vol. 24: *Correspondence, dispatches, reports, ordinances, memoranda and other papers relating to the affairs of Hong Kong, 1846–60* (Shannon: Irish University Press, 1971), 109–150.
6 G. B. Endacott, *A History of Hong Kong.* Revised edition (Hong Kong: Oxford University Press, 1973), 77–78.
7 T. N. Chiu, *The Port of Hong Kong: A survey of its development* (Hong Kong: Hong Kong University Press, 1973), 32–36.
8 Endacott, *A History of Hong Kong*, 276.
9 Ng Lun Ngai Ha, *Interactions of East and West: Development of Public Education in Early Hong Kong* (Hong Kong: The Chinese University Press, 1983).
10 Dafydd Emrys Evans, "Chinatown in Hong Kong: The beginnings of Taiping-shan,"*Journal of the Hong Kong Branch of the Royal Asiatic Society*, 10 (1970), 68–78.
11 Figures from *Hong Kong Blue Books* for the respective years.
12 Government Notice No. 57, *Hong Kong Government Gazette* (May 10, 1856).
13 Statement by Governor William Robinson, as quoted in Pryor, "The Great plague of Hong Kong," 65.
14 David Faure, *A Documentary History of Hong Kong: Society* (Hong Kong: Hong Kong University Press, 2003), 47.
15 For details of this Ordinance, see "An Ordinance for Reservation of a European District in the City of Victoria (amended)," *Hong Kong Government Gazette* (April 21, 1888), 375–376.

16 *Council Sitting Record of Legislative Council of Hong Kong, Legislative Council of Hong Kong,* March 28, 1904.

17 David Faure, "The common people in Hong Kong history," in Lee Pui Tak ed., *Colonial Hong Kong and Modern China: Interaction and Reintegration* (Hong Kong: Hong Kong University Press, 2005), 15.

18 Endacott, *A History of Hong Kong,* 115.

19 Anthony Hedley, "The role of public health in social justice: the next steps in Hong Kong," in Gabriel M. Leung and John Bacon-Shone eds., *Hong Kong's Health System: Reflections, Perspectives and Visions* (Hong Kong: Hong Kong University Press, 2006), 118–119. See also Ian Morley, "City chaos, contagion, and social justice," *Yale Journal of Biology and Medicine,* 80:2 (June 2007), 61–72.

20 Faure, *A Documentary History of Hong Kong: Society,* 46.

21 Gerald Choa, *The Life and Times of Sir Kai Ho Kai,* 2nd ed. (Hong Kong: Chinese University Press, 2000), 89–91.

22 For a biography of Ho, see Choa, *The Life and Times of Sir Kai Ho Kai.*

23 Faure, *A Documentary History of Hong Kong: Society,* 86–88.

24 Lau Siu Kai, *Society and Politics in Hong Kong* (Hong Kong: Chinese University Press, 1982), 48.

25 *Historical and Statistical Abstract of the Colony of Hong Kong.* 2nd ed. (Hong Kong: Hong Kong Government, 1911) Historical Part, 2.

26 Yip, "Colonialism, disease, and public health: malaria in the history of Hong Kong," 12.

27 "Colonial Surgeon's Report for 1877," *The Hong Kong Government Gazette, 6 July, 1878,* 330.

28 "The Colonial Surgeon's Report for 1851," *Hong Kong Administrative Reports* (Hong Kong: Government Printers, 1852).

29 Starling et al., *Plague, SARS and the Story of Medicine in Hong Kong,* 23.

30 Ka-che Yip, "Science, culture, and disease control in colonial Hong Kong," in Liping Bu, Darwin H. Stapleton, and Ka-che Yip eds., *Science, Public Health and the State in Modern Asia* (London: Routledge, 2012), 25–26.

31 Ka-che Yip, "Segregation, isolation, and quarantine: protecting Hong Kong from diseases in the pre-war period," *Journal of Contemporary Asian Development,* 11:1 (June 2012), 93–116.

32 Ordinance 12 of 1857, *Hong Kong Government Gazette* (November 28, 1857).

33 Levine, "Modernity, Medicine, and Colonialism," 676–677.

34 The reports have been reprinted in *China,* Vol. 25: *Correspondence, dispatches, reports, returns memorials and other papers respecting the affairs of Hong Kong, 1862–81* (Shannon: Irish University Press, 1971), 506–639.

35 *Lord Kimberley's Defence of the Government Brothel System at Hong Kong: Correspondence Relating to the Contagious Ordinances in Hong Kong* (London: National Association for the Appeal of the Contagious Diseases Act, 1882).

36 Starling et al. *Plague, SARS and the Story of Medicine in Hong Kong,* 85–88.

37 H. A. Rydings, "Transactions of the China Medico-Chirurgical Society, 1845–6," *Journal of the Hong Kong Branch of the Royal Asiatic Society,* 13 (1973): 13–27.

38 Hui Po Keung, "Comprador politics and middlemen capitalism," in Ngo Tak-wing ed., *Hong Kong's History: State and Society under Colonial Rule* (London: Routledge, 1999), 36.

39 Sinn, *Power and Charity: The Early History of the Tung Wah Hospital;* and Hutcheon, *Bedside Manner,* 12. A team of historians from the Chinese University of Hong Kong has assembled and published a five-volume collection of key documents about the Tung Wah Hospital entitled, *Donghua Sanyuan danan ziliao huibian xilie* [Collection of archival materials about the Tung Wah Hospitals] (Hong Kong: Joint Publishing Company, 2009–2010).

40 G. H. Choa, "The Lowson diary: a record of the early phase of the Hong Kong bubonic plague 1894," *Journal of the Royal Asiatic Society Hong Kong Branch*, 33 (1993), 129–145.
41 "Medical Report on the Epidemic of Bubonic Plague in 1894," *Hong Kong Legislative Council Sessional Papers, 2 March 1895* (Hong Kong: Government Printers, 1895).
42 Choa, *The Life and Times of Sir Kai Ho Kai*, 279.
43 Tom Solomon, "Hong Kong, 1894: the role of James A Lowson in the controversial discovery of the plague bacillus," *The Lancet*, 350 (1997), 59–62. See also Bjorn P. Zietz and Hartmut Dunkelberg, "The history of the plague and the research on the causative agent *Yersinia Pestis*," *International Journal of Hygiene and Environmental Health*, 207 (2004), 165–178.
44 Echenberg, *Plague Ports*, 43.
45 Y. W. Lau, *A History of the Municipal Councils of Hong Kong 1883–1999: From the Sanitary Board to the Urban Council and the Regional Council* (Hong Kong: Leisure and Cultural Services Department, 2002), 61–62; and Shiona Airlie, *Thistle and Bamboo: The Life and Times of Sir James Stewart Lockhart* (Hong Kong: Oxford University Press, 1989).
46 Law, "Xifang yixue yu zhimin guanzhi yi erci shijie dazhan qian Xianggang he Xinjiapo wei bijiao gean," 134.
47 Sinn, *Power and Charity*.
48 Endacott, *A History of Hong Kong*, 217; and Pryor, "The great plague of Hong Kong," 64.

3 Disease, scientific medicine, and public health

From the plague epidemic to the early twentieth century

At the turn of the century, Hong Kong was very much affected by the tumultuous changes taking place in China, and these developments once again reflected the importance of the "China factor" in Hong Kong's history. The fortunes of the declining Qing dynasty reached a nadir when it was defeated by Japan in 1895. Japan's victory marked the beginning of a "scramble for concessions" in China by the major powers, and one of Britain's demands was the extension of Hong Kong's boundaries to China's border that resulted in Britain's leasing of the New Territories in 1898 for 99 years. This enabled the dispersal of the growing population, as well as the burgeoning manufacturing industries to the largely rural territory. The extension of control inevitably meant the need to expand public health and medical care to protect the population and labor force in areas that were still lacking in essential sanitary and medical support. Another step bringing Hong Kong closer to China occurred in 1912 when the Kowloon–Canton railway opened, thereby facilitating the movement of people, goods, and, with increased traffic, the spread of pathogens between the colony and the mainland. Indeed, these developments proved critical in the future spread of diseases, and would alert health authorities on both sides of the border to the need for regional cooperation to combat epidemics.

The Revolution of 1911 in China led to the downfall of the Qing and the founding of the Republic of China. Hong Kong had been used as a base by anti-Manchu revolutionaries, and among the conspirators was Dr. Sun Yat-sen, the founder of the Republic of China. In 1892, Sun graduated from the Hong Kong College of Medicine for Chinese, founded in 1887. In that same year, Alice Memorial Hospital was opened with a donation from Dr. Ho Kai, a member of the colony's Chinese elite, and the hospital provided facilities for the students' clinical study.

These developments reflected the changing landscape of medical training in Hong Kong, and indeed, in the world of medical science as a whole. The discovery of plague bacillus by Dr. Shibasaburo Kitasato and Dr. Alexandre Yersin in 1894 brought considerable excitement among physicians and medical researchers in Hong Kong and beyond. In the West, the rise of the germ theory and the association of medicine with the laboratory had revolutionized the understanding of disease causation and the training of physicians. In Hong Kong, institutional developments at the turn of the century reflected, to a significant extent, the impact of scientific medicine. These changes included the founding of the Hong Kong College of Medicine for Chinese in 1887, the Bacteriological Institute in 1906, and the Faculty of Medicine at the University of Hong Kong in 1912. At the same time, a new understanding of the etiology of diseases led to changes in health policies and disease-control strategies. This chapter examines the institutionalization of scientific medicine in Hong Kong and how scientific medicine impacted the colonial government's formulation and implementation of control measures against such diseases as plague, beriberi, malaria, and tuberculosis.

Scientific medicine and public health

The rise of scientific medicine in the nineteenth century led to a paradigm shift in the practice of medicine in the West. Andrew Cunningham and Perry Williams have classified the changes of medical paradigms over time: from "bedside medicine (from the Middle Ages to the 18th century)," to "hospital medicine (from late-18th century to mid-19th century)," and to "laboratory medicine (from the later part of the 19th century to the present)."[1] Advancements in laboratory medicine depended on the technological development of the microscope which enabled physicians and scientists to observe the disease processes at their cellular level, paving the way for the emergence of what became known as cellular pathology.[2] Researchers like Rudolf Virchow, Robert Koch, and Louis Pasteur, contributed to innovations and new procedures in medicine and the rise of the "germ theory" of disease. Koch, for example, discovered the causal organisms of tuberculosis and cholera, and scientists and physicians employing similar research techniques and procedures helped to lay the foundation for the new discipline of bacteriology. The laboratory revolution also transformed medical education, with universities in Europe and North America playing an increasingly significant role in scientific medical research. By the 1920s, "the university teaching of medicine had become the standard in much of Europe and was almost unchallenged as a goal in the United States and, to a lesser extent, in Britain. This fusion of laboratory medicine with clinic in a university setting proved to be the key development in the shaping of twentieth century medical education."[3]

The rise of scientific medicine had far-reaching consequences for the development of public health. Unlike the sanitary and environmental movements that had dominated public health approaches, the germ theory reoriented the attention to the individual, and physicians or medical experts, rather than engineers and sanitarians, began to play an increasingly important role in the formulation of health and disease-control policies. In the name of protecting the public's health and improving the quality of life, the state became more interventionist in instituting such mandatory measures as vaccinations or imposing regulations to control infectious diseases. Certainly, the emphasis on the strictly medical aspects of public health did not mean the end of sanitary and environmental reforms, especially when research required heavy investments in institution building and the training of personnel. In some cases, as in the efforts to control malaria in Hong Kong, a combination of approaches proved to be more practical and economical as far as the government was concerned.

Institutionalizing scientific medicine in Hong Kong

The laboratory-based germ theory of diseases also proved to be important in "establishing the basis of disease-management in the colonies of the European imperial powers at the end of nineteenth century, and in shaping modern attitudes to cleanliness and hygiene."[4] It would be difficult to exactly date the transition in Hong Kong from "hospital medicine" to "laboratory medicine," but by the turn of the century, several events marked the beginning of significant developments in hospital care and education, including the opening of the Alice Memorial Hospital in 1887 and the Hong Kong College of Medicine for Chinese.[5] Members of the hospital staff served as instructors in the College of Medicine while the hospital itself provided facilities for the students' clinical study. Managed by the London Missionary Society, the hospital was the first hospital to train local Chinese in Western medicine.

One of the founders of the medical college was Dr. Patrick Manson, the famous parasitologist who was later honored as the "Father of Tropical Medicine." Manson had worked for the Chinese Imperial Maritime Customs in Amoy and was also a well-respected physician along coastal China. His research had led to the discovery that filariasis in humans was transmitted by mosquitoes. At the opening of the college, Manson assured the public that the college could serve a purpose of turning Hong Kong into "a centre of light and guidance to China in all matters pertaining to civilization."[6] He thought Hong Kong a better place for the founding of a medical college for the Chinese because there were competent students whose skills and knowledge in the English language enabled them to grasp the latest medical knowledge.[7] Yet, there were personnel and operational problems that hampered the development of the college. First, there was tension between medical missionaries and other physicians associated with the hospital and the college. According to some contemporary accounts, Manson himself apparently had difficulties working with the medical mission in Amoy during the 1870s. The college depended heavily on part-time lecturers who also engaged in private practice. They did not necessarily share a common philosophy regarding the management of the hospital and the college in general, and healing approaches in particular.[8] Moreover, the research culture in the college was only of a rudimentary level, although some were active in their own research. Dr. James Cantlie, a founder of the College, did most of his research in the hospital on the Peak that he established. John Thomson, a medical missionary working in both the hospital and the college, engaged in malaria research funded by the government. But his results were overlooked in the official report by the special committee on malaria appointed by the Hong Kong government.[9] Finally, the attempt to have its graduates recognized by the British Medical Council was vigorously pursued yet unsuccessful.[10] Employment opportunities for graduates were therefore limited. The Hong Kong government hired one "Chinese Medical Officer" in 1899 as the only resident physician to take care of the New Territories.[11] In 1902, four more "Chinese Medical Officers" were appointed: one in charge of the General Dispensary, one as the Laboratory Assistant, and two as Bacteriologist Assistants.[12] Most graduates moved out of Hong Kong to search for employment opportunities elsewhere. The college closed in 1915, having produced 51 graduates in its 23 years of existence.

Another major step in the development of scientific medicine was the appointment of a bacteriologist by the government in 1902 and subsequently the founding in 1906 of the Bacteriological Institute to serve as a center for research and disease control. The recurring outbreaks of plague after 1894 had adversely affected Hong Kong as it disrupted trade and the movement of goods and people. In 1901, the Hong Kong government initiated the process of creating a new position for Bacteriologist within the civil service. At first, London's reaction was negative because the position was regarded redundant as similar personnel and facilities had been established in India, Kula Lumpur, and other parts of the British Empire in Asia. Fortunately, Patrick Manson's intervention proved decisive. In 1889, Manson left Hong Kong for Britain where he continued medical practice and research. The Colonial Office appointed him medical adviser, offering expert opinions on matters relating to tropical diseases in Asia and Africa. Manson supported the proposal from the Hong Kong government and recommended Dr. William Hunter to fill the post. A top graduate in 1893 from the University of Aberdeen, Hunter furthered his studies in Berlin in pathology and bacteriology. Prior to his Hong Kong appointment, he was the director of the Pathological Institute of the London Hospital. Young and ambitious, he aspired to break new grounds in the study of tropical disease.[13] He successfully negotiated for better laboratory equipment, and started in biomedical research, especially on plague control and prevention, once he arrived in Hong Kong in 1902.[14] He held two other concurrent appointments as the superintendent of the Government Vaccine Institute and that of the government public mortuary.[15] Outside of the government, he was a lecturer in Pathology and Bacteriology at the Hong Kong College of Medicine for Chinese. In 1906, a modern laboratory was eventually built and furnished, thereby providing significant support for pathological investigations into the causes of disease and epidemic.[16] In 1909, Hunter passed away after he was infected while doing research. He was succeeded by Harold MacFarlane who took up almost all positions left by Hunter, including the teaching duties at the Hong Kong College of Medicine and then University of Hong Kong (HKU) until 1919 when he died.[17] The Bacteriological Institute proved to be a major step forward in Hong Kong's attempt to control infectious diseases as it began a diagnostic and infectious disease surveillance service for the colony.

The most important impetus for the institutionalization of scientific medicine was the founding of the Faculty of Medicine at HKU in 1912. Governor Frederick Lugard was the chief architect behind the founding of the university and had a vision for the development of a medical faculty.[18] As a university, the question of full recognition for medical graduates was no longer a problem. Yet, the transition from the medical college into medical faculty was not easy as the newly founded university did not award college graduates degrees *ad eundem*.[19] A considerable number of graduates and former students from the College of Medicine enrolled and completed their medical training at the newly founded HKU. The very first HKU graduate was Dr. George Harold Thomas, a graduate from the Hong Kong College of Medicine. Between 1914 and 1942, the number of graduates totaled 365, meaning that an average of slightly more than a dozen of medical graduates were produced annually over these years.[20] Although the university did not have a large number of full-time teaching members, it was a marked improvement from the conditions at the Hong Kong College of Medicine. They could focus more on teaching and, more importantly, build up the medical faculty through the cultivation of research culture in scientific medicine. To pursue this goal, Kenelm H. Digby, a leader of the medical faculty before WWII,[21] remarked in 1919, "[t]his university is in its early childhood; it will not have fully established its title till it produces original research of value."[22] To realize this objective, HKU's medical society edited and published its journal, *The Caduceus: Journal of the Hong Kong University Medical Society*. As in the case of the *Lancet*, for example, the journal would serve as an important device for the spread of latest research and discussions about the practice of medicine.[23] In fact, a study shows that between 1914 and 1941, chair professors at HKU's medical faculty published a total of 174 papers in leading medical journals, of which 81 percent were either in the *British Medical Journal* or the *Lancet*.[24]

The plagues and rats

The discovery of the plague bacillus in 1894 was only the beginning of a long journey in combating the plague. In 1896, there was an outbreak of plague with 1,204 cases recorded, and the mortality rate was 89.5 percent. A physician seconded from the German East Asia Squadron (*Ostasiengeschwader*), Dr. M Wilm took charge of the Kennedy Town Hospital, the plague hospital. He thus had access to specimen and collected substantial information from post-mortem examinations. His research report was received by the Legislative Council,[25] and Governor Robinson praised his contributions and hoped that his research would "prove of much benefit in dealing with this terrible disease."[26]

Robinson's successor Henry Blake had a strong interest in scientific medicine, and was certainly concerned with the persistent problem of plague[27] Between 1898 and 1901, the average annual number of plague cases was 1,378 and the average mortality rate remained high at 94.35 percent.[28] Furthermore, Hong Kong and London were at odds as to whether or not infected individuals should be allowed to leave Hong Kong for their homeland in South China. The Colonial Office in London maintained that Hong Kong had to comply with the international Venice convention banning the export of diseases. Governor Blake, however, wanted support from medical authorities to legitimize the prevailing practice, and in 1901, with backing from both the Executive and Legislative councils, he pressed London for support. In the meantime, Blake solicited expert opinions from public health and tropical diseases authorities for plague prevention recommendations, and also planned to hire a bacteriologist to carry on laboratory investigation into the plague and other prevailing diseases and epidemics. London subsequently sent Obsert Chadwick and Dr. William J. R Simpson to advise the governor on plague control. This was Chadwick's third visit to Hong Kong since the early 1880s, and he proposed plans to improve water supply and sewerage and drainage systems from the perspective of a sanitarian and engineer.[29] Dr. Simpson had worked in Asia and Africa before he was appointed professor of hygiene at King's College, London, and he moved to the London School of Tropical Medicine at its founding. He spent the first seven months of 1902 in Hong Kong. His research confirmed the role of rats in the transmission of the plague, and through the help of the government bacteriologist and his assistants, Simpson established the high correlation pattern between infected rats and the spread of plague among people in the community. He supported the rat eradication campaigns and microscopic analysis of dead rats to identify any potential outbreaks. The most important recommendation for Blake, however, was perhaps his support of the government's position on the question of free movement of infected patients and bodies to South China. In other words, he believed that stipulations in the Venice Convention did not fit the local and regional circumstances within Hong Kong and South China.[30] Simpson's recommendations were implemented by the government, and "every dead or sick rat in the colony" would be examined bacteriologically, and when plague was confirmed in a locality, preventive measures would be put in place immediately.[31] Scientific medicine played a key role in informing and shaping the government's public health policies.

The study of the etiology of plague was continued by Dr. William Hunter who headed the Bacteriological Institute. His 150-page report was by far the most comprehensive research into the plague at that time and it revealed the dynamic interactions among those conducting scientific medical research in plague.[32] He was meticulous in his research procedures, and he distinguished between two major types of plague, namely *plague septicemia* and *primary plague pneumonia*, to each of which he gave pathological and clinical description.[33] But as he had focused on contaminated food as a possible source of infection, echoing observations made by several other researchers, "examination of rats for fleas and flea counts was therefore not performed initially."[34] In 1898, French navy doctor Paul–Louis Simond, working in

India, demonstrated that the flea was the vector for the plague, a discovery that was confirmed later by other scientists.

The anti-plague measures that the Hong Kong government adopted focused on rat eradication campaigns and the examination of infected rats. The government encouraged residents to prevent intrusion of rats by installing iron railings at drain and ventilation openings, and the destruction of rats by poison and traps. All dead rats were collected for bacteriological examination. At least once every three months, systematic cleansing and washing of all native dwellings with a flea-killing mixture as well as daily removal of trash from all houses and scavenging of streets were carried out. Finally, plague-infested premises, including household furniture, were disinfected and washed thoroughly. What is significant was that these measures were not only implemented in Hong Kong island and Kowloon, but also in the New Territories as its population had been growing by the turn of the century.[35]

Tuberculosis and malaria

Scientific medical research also played a role in the long struggle against such prevalent infectious diseases as tuberculosis and malaria. As noted in the previous chapter, tuberculosis, although a threat to people's health, was not considered to be a pressing health problem by the Hong Kong government. Before 1882 when the German bacteriologist Robert Koch discovered the tubercle bacillus as the cause of the disease, tuberculosis was generally associated with filth and impure air. Although Koch's discovery did not lead to a cure of the disease, a substance prepared from the proteins of the tubercle bacillus proved to be an effective diagnostic tool – the tuberculin skin test. That, coupled with the discovery of the X-ray in 1895, made mass screening for the disease possible in the early half of the twentieth century.[36] In 1920, two French scientists developed the BCG (bacilli calmette Guerin) vaccine, but it was not widely used until after World War II.

The mortality rate of tuberculosis remained high by the turn of the century. In 1906, tuberculosis recorded the highest percentage, 11 percent, of total deaths for that year, and it remained within the top three diseases claiming most lives during the 1910s and early 1920s.[37] What is significant is that in 1897, the Colonial Surgeon had already identified the cause of the high mortality from tuberculosis as "overcrowding, inefficient ventilation and poverty."[38] That being the case, the logical conclusion would be for the government to initiate reforms to alleviate those problems. Certainly, there were additional attempts to improve housing conditions, but the government was not ready to push for more radical and fundamental reforms in social and working conditions, as such efforts would make the government and industry largely financially responsible for the control of the disease. The thrust of the anti-tuberculosis effort was directed instead toward correcting individual behavior, since the disease could be transmitted by individual actions such as sneezing, coughing, or spitting. Hence, education, monitoring, and prohibiting spitting – the "uncivilized" and "disgusting" habit of most Chinese – became the main thrust of the policy in controlling the disease. When the Legislative Council debated the passage of an anti-spitting bill in 1908, the representative from the Chamber of Commerce proclaimed that trying to educate the Chinese on the evils of spitting was a waste of time, and that the government was correct in legislating proper behavior so that people realized that they "must not spit promiscuously where they please."[39] In the name of public health, the government was intervening in people's life and prescribing rules of behavior. Ironically, Henry H. Scott, government bacteriologist echoed the government's claim to protecting the public's health while arriving at a different conclusion when he wrote in 1921 that the problems of tuberculosis in Hong Kong were "really social problems, and are, therefore, intimately connected with those of public health."[40]

The government's anti-malaria policy reflected to a significant extent, the same reluctance of the government to fund costly infrastructural improvements. Yet in the case of malaria, the hitherto approach, based on the linkage of the disease to filth and foul air and the control thereof with sanitary improvements, had succeeded to some extent in spite of the ignorance of the scientific fact that such improvements had helped to suppress mosquitoes that later were identified as the vector of the disease. By 1898, the research of Patrick Manson, Ronald Ross, Giovanni Battista, and others had identified the mosquito as the malaria vector, thereby offering a new vector-centered approach in the struggle against malaria. Certainly, after the plague epidemic of 1894, there was a sense of urgency on the part of the government to introduce reforms to ensure Hong Kong's health. The vector control strategy actually was less costly than large-scale public health improvements and could in fact be based on the expansion and refinement of the sanitary and environmental approach that had been in place already.

In 1899, a broad anti-malaria campaign was initiated, the thrust of which was to control the breeding of mosquitoes and the destruction of the vector. Larval breeding places were located and destroyed, and standing water was treated with kerosene or carbolated creosote. Proper nullah drainage and elimination of larval breeding grounds became the main focus of the campaign. Public health education programs directed at school children and the public were carried out to publicize the scientific facts of infection by mosquitoes and the methods of mosquito control and destruction. The government even administered quinine to school children in selected districts. To monitor the spread of the disease and maintain surveillance, the Medical Officer of Health received weekly reports of all malaria cases from hospitals. The Bacteriological Institute also conducted scientific studies of malaria and mosquito species, and results were sent to the Imperial Bureau of Entomology in London. Malaria mortality remained at an average of 431 per annum from 1900 to 1904, and 378 from 1910 to 1914, but significantly, there was a reduction of almost 60 percent of malaria deaths from 1910 to 1914. Yet, malarial infection remained rife in the New Territories, and the government resorted to prophylactic injections of quinine in certain areas as well as to the Chinese staff of the Kowloon–Canton Railway.[41]

Beriberi and nutrition

Beriberi is a nutritional disorder caused by a deficiency of vitamin B1 (thiamine); the consequence can be deadly because it often leads to heart failure.[42] It is now known that the prevalence of beriberi was a result of the use of steam-powered machines in dehusking rice since the mid-1850s.[43] The zenith of European colonialism in nineteenth-century Asia paved the way for a sophisticated trade network by which commodities were now more accessible in different parts of Asia. Rice, the major staple food in Asia, was one of such commodities. Efficiency in the process of rice milling by steamed-power machines lowered the nutritional value of rice.

Initially, researchers looking for a cause of the disease were misled by the germ theory paradigm which dominated scientific medical thinking at the turn of the century.[44] Since the mid-nineteenth century, beriberi had caused much concern among countries and colonies in Asia. In Hong Kong, Dr. Ho Kai was probably one of the earliest to become interested in finding a solution to the problem. Writing on the development of beriberi in the Philippines, Dr. Arthur J. Jefferson, a medical officer of Rochale infirmary, had described his meeting with Ho Kai in December 1888, in which he learned of the efforts of their former classmate Mr. Kanehiro Takaki, who had allegedly stamped out beriberi from the Japanese navy by the introduction of a more nitrogenous dietary. However, Ho Kai argued that "absolute immunity was not... to be obtained merely by the liberal indulgence in nitrogenous food, nor with the Britisher to be regarded as being exempt from the disease."[45]

In Hong Kong, the number of deaths caused by beriberi during the two decades from 1891 to 1910 was alarming: they ranged from 128 in 1891 to 377 in 1900, and from 676 in 1905 to 562 in 1910.[46] Dr. James Cantile, Dean of Hong Kong College of Medicine for Chinese made a major effort in promoting an understanding of the disease when he translated a study of the disease in 1893. He had hoped that his interest in studies of beriberi in the Dutch East Indies, India, Japan, and Singapore would help him identify causes and remedies for the growing number of such cases at the Alice Memorial Hospital in Hong Kong.[47] The first scientific study of beriberi was conducted by Dr. Robert McLean Gibosn, medical superintendent of the Alice Memorial Hospital and a part-time teaching faculty at the Hong Kong College of Medicine for Chinese.[48] His study pointed to a substantial difference in the number of male and female patients: the average ratio of men and women patients was 22:1 between 1888 and 1899. Moreover, Gibson identified the poorer class as more likely to develop beriberi. The difference in male and female morbidity, however, was more a result of the gender structure in late nineteenth-century Hong Kong than differences in physical conditions between men and women. Most Chinese immigrants were male and they did not bring their families to Hong Kong until they found a rather secure job. In other words, the chance for women suffering from deficiency in nutrition was lower than that of men.

As to the causes of the disease, the prevailing theory was based on Patrick Manson's argument that it was a result of "chemical poison generated by a bacterium which resides in the soil in fomites." The argument was repeated by Dr. Francis William Clark, the Medical Officer of the Hong Kong government and a part-time lecturer of the Hong Kong College of Medicine for Chinese, Ronald Ross, and others, although some physicians suggested that the disease was caused by moldy rice, or transmitted by an unknown vector.

The research of the bacteriologist William Hunter, however, led him to different conclusions from many of his contemporaries, especially those of Hamilton Wright, who set up the Pathological Institute in Kuala Lumpur in 1902.[49] Hunter pointed out that in his research, there was "no evidence of a primary lesion," by which "virus entered into the body." Also, "no specific micro-organisms" were discovered in any part of the patients' bodies; finally, he found out that it was impossible to induce beriberi in any of the animals (monkeys, pigs, sheep, calves, rabbits, and fowls) that he used for the experiments. As a result, he did not consider beriberi "a highly infectious disease," and concluded that the correct treatment was to provide patients with "a liberal and wholesome diet" in a room of good ventilation – a course of action that proved to be correct later.[50]

Hunter buttressed his case by showing how his conclusions benefitted the colonial government economically. Specially, he pointed out that "a disease, occurring as it does in human beings during the most strenuous and wage-earning period of life, becomes of serious importance in a community like our own, where our commercial prosperity is largely dependent on the momentum for labour bestowed on it by the Chinese coolie who, unfortunately, is only too frequently its victim."[51] In his statistical data on the patients' occupational background, there were 2,907 cases, out of which 1,735 were coolies. Of the 1,735 cases, 857 died.[52]

Hunter's views were basically endorsed by the physicians who attended the conference of the Far Eastern Association of Tropical Medicine held in Manila in March 1910. They passed a resolution declaring that "in the opinion of this association, sufficient evidence has now been produced in support of the view that beriberi is associated with the continuous consumption of white (polished) rice as the staple article of diet, and the association accordingly desires to bring this matter to the notice of the various Governments concerned."[53]

The Hong Kong government responded to the resolution with its usual laissez faire manner. Since beriberi was not caused by bacteria, it thus had no place in the work of the government bacteriologist. In fact, further research on beriberi did not fit into any of the government's research establishment. Moreover, beriberi was not a disease that could make Hong Kong an "infected port." On February 24, 1911, Cecil Clementi, the Colonial Secretary, issued the following notification,

The attention of all persons who consume white rice and also of all large employers of coolie labour is directed to the fact that it is generally believed that the disease Beri-beri, which causes several hundred deaths in Hong Kong each year, is produced by the consumption of white rice, as the staple article of diet, without a sufficiency of other foods.

It is important therefore that a sufficient quantity of fresh fish should be eaten with the rice, but if this cannot be afforded beans should be eaten, in the proportion of not less than one quarter of a catty of beans to every catty of rice. The beans should be boiled with a small quantity of fresh pork or fresh fish to make a soup.[54]

The recommendation was not mandatory, nor was it enforced by any legislation. Apart from circulating the recommendation to all large employers of Chinese laborers, the Hong Kong government did not carry out any further action regarding the disease until the late 1930s.[55]

The health of Hong Kong

By the turn of the century, the health of Hong Kong remained rather poor although it had gradually recovered from the plague epidemic. With 2,146 cases, the incidence of plague was severe in 1914. In that same year, 769 persons died from tuberculosis, 241 from malaria, and 399 from beriberi. The death rate for the population actually had increased slightly from 22.3 per 1,000 in 1899 to 23.34 per 1,000 in 1914. According to health officials, the health conditions in Hong Kong in the early 1910s were very much affected by the increases in incidence of infectious diseases in the New Territories, as well as the continual influx of migrants from China, especially during the political turmoil after the fall of the Qing.[56] The overcrowded conditions in the Chinese quarters continued to be a major problem despite the passage of ordinances in 1894 to improve the housing situation. Another ordinance, the Public Health and Buildings Ordinance was passed in 1903 after the investigation of Simpson and Chadwick had exposed the lack of improvements in general housing conditions. There were now stipulations about open spaces and scavenging lanes as well as specifications for the height and types of buildings. The interior divisions of dwellings were required to ensure adequate light and ventilation for the rooms. The ordinance remained the major piece of legislation governing housing in the colony until 1935. However, with the continued growth of industries in the colony during the interwar period and the proliferation of small family workshops in the congested Chinese tenements, living as well as health conditions for the poor and workers would actually deteriorate despite general improvements in living standards. The next chapter will examine the government's public health and medical care policies during a time of rapid industrialization in the interwar years, and how the Japanese occupation affected the health infrastructure and services.

Notes

1 "Introduction," Andrew Cunningham and Perry Williams, ed., *The Laboratory Revolution in Medicine* (New York: Cambridge University Press, 2002), 1–2.
2 Mark Harrison, *Disease and the Modern World: 1500 to the Present Day* (Cambridge: Polity Press, 2008), 118–122.
3 Thomas N. Bonner, *Becoming a Physician: Medical Education in Britain, France, Germany and the United States, 1750–1945* (New York: Oxford University Press, 1995), 288.
4 Ibid., 4–5.
5 For details, see Timothy Man Kong Wong, "Local Voluntarism: The Medical Mission of the London Missionary Society in Nineteenth Century China," David Hardiman ed., *Healing Bodies, Saving Souls: Medical Missions in Asia and Africa* (The Wellcome Series in the History of Medicine, Clio Media 80) (Amsterdam: Rodopi, 2006), 87–113.
6 "Inauguration of the Medical College: Public Meeting in Hong Kong- The Inaugural Addresses," *China Mail* (October 1, 1887).
7 Li Shangren, *Diguo de yshi: Wanbade yu Yingguoredai yixue de chuangjian* [Physician of the empire: Manson and the creation of British tropical medicine] (Taibei: Yunchen wenhuashiye gufen youxian gongxi, 2012), 213.
8 Peter Cunich, *A History of the University of Hong Kong. Vol. 1: 1911–1945* (Hong Kong: Hong Kong University Press, 2012), 52–64.
9 Ibid., 65.
10 See, Law, "Xifang yixue yu Zhimin Guanzhi: yi Erci Shijie Dazhan qian Xianggang he Xinjiapo wei Bijiao Gean," 172–180.
11 *The Blue Book of the Hong Kong Government for the Year of 1899*, I74.
12 *The Blue Book of the Hong Kong Government for the Year of 1902*, J96–J97.
13 "Death of Dr. William Hunter, Government Bacteriologist," *The British Medical Journal*, 2534 (July 24, 1909), 238.
14 Starling et al., *Plague, SARS and the Story of Medicine in Hong Kong*, 147–224.
15 His date of report to duty was February 27, 1902. On October 15, 1902, he was joined by Dr Ho Ko Tsun in the capacity of Laboratory Assistant, and Dr Lee Yin See as well as Dr Chan Fai Kwong in the capacity of Bacteriologist Assistants. See, *The Blue Book of the Hong Kong Government for the Year of 1902*, J96–J97.
16 For details about the design and layout of the building, see Starling et al. *Plague, SARS and the Story of Medicine in Hong Kong*, 158–160.
17 Dafydd Evans, *Constancy of Purpose: An Account of the Foundation and History of the Hong Kong College of Medicine and the Faculty of Medicine of the University of Hong Kong, 1887–1987* (Hong Kong: Hong Kong University Press, 1987), 262.
18 Chan Lau Kit-ching and Peter Cunich eds., *An Impossible Dream: Hong Kong University from Foundation to Re-establishment, 1910–1950* (New York: Oxford University Press, 2002), 1–23.
19 Cunich, *A History of the University of Hong Kong,* 72–73.
20 Starling et al., *Plague, SARS and the Story of Medicine in Hong Kong*, 342.
21 Digby was the most important staff on the HKU medical faculty before 1945. He served in a number of significant capacities: Chair of Surgery (1915–1945), Chair of Anatomy (1913–) and Dean of Medicine for three terms of office (1915–1916, 1920–1922, and 1923–1925). For details of his life, see Julia L. Y. Chan and N. G. Patil, *Digby: A Remarkable Life* (Hong Kong: Hong Kong University Press, 2006).
22 "The Objects of a Medical Society: An abstract of address delivered before the Medical Society in September 1919," *The Caduceus: Journal of the Hong Kong University Medical Society*, 1:1 (April 1922): 20–21.
23 W. H. Mcmenemey, "Medical History: The Lancet, 1823–1973," *British Medical Journal*, 5882 (September 29, 1973): 680–684. See also, Jim Garner, "*The Lancet*

celebrates 150th anniversary, still following its founder's footsteps," *Canadian Medical Association Journal*, 109 (December 15, 1973): 1254–1255.

24 For a general discussion of the emergence of research culture in medicine in Hong Kong, see Timothy Man Kong Wong, "Higher Education and Research Culture in Hong Kong: With Special Reference to Medical Education, Research and Professionalism, 1880s-1980s," in Ricardo Mak ed., *Transmitting the Ideal of Enlightenment: Chinese Universities since the Nineteenth Century* (Lanham: University Press of America, 2009), 83–108.

25 "Report of the Plague," *Sessional Paper for the Year of 1896*, 296–271.

26 Minutes of Proceedings of the Legislative Council, *The Hong Kong Hansard* (December 3, 1896): 6.

27 Mary Preston Sutphen, "Imperial Hygiene in Calcutta, Cape Town, and Hong Kong: The Early Career of Sir Wiliam John Ritchie Simpson (1855–1931)." Ph.D. thesis, Yale University (1995), 348–356.

28 The average numbers are calculated from the figures provided by Choa, *The Life and Times of Sir Kai Ho Kai*, 278.

29 In particular, he made numerous proposals for sewers and drainage improvements. For details, see Lau, *A History of the Municipal Councils of Hong Kong 1883–1999*, 65–66.

30 Simpson's reports were presented to the Legislative Council, and thus collected in the Sessional Papers of 1902. See Sutphen, "Imperial Hygiene in Calcutta, Cape Town, and Hong Kong," 381–407.

31 Ibid., 399.

32 William Hunter, *A Research into the Epidemic and Epizootic Plague* (Hong Kong: Hong Kong Government, 1904).

33 Ibid., 544.

34 Starling et al., *Plague, SARS and the Story of Medicine in Hong Kong*, 163.

35 *Medical and Sanitary Reports for the Year 1914*, 24–25.

36 Kenneth F. Kiple, *The Cambridge World History of Human Disease* (Cambridge: Cambridge University Press, 1993), 1064–1065.

37 Margaret Jones, "Tuberculosis, Housing and the colonial state: Hong Kong, 1900–1950," *Modern Asian Studies*, 37:3 (July 2003), 663.

38 *Report of the Medical Officer of Health, the Sanitary Surveyor, and the Colonial Veterinary Surgeon for the year 1897*, 274.

39 *Minutes of the Legislative Council, 10th December, 1908.*

40 Henry H. Scott, "The prevalence and character of tuberculosis in Hong Kong," *Annals of Tropical Medicine and Parasitology*, 15 (1921), 213.

41 *Medical and Sanitary Reports for the Year 1914*, 20–21, 62–63. See also Yip, "Colonialism, disease, and public health: malaria in the history of Hong Kong," 18–20.

42 E. A. Martin ed., *Concise Medical Dictionary.* 8 ed. (Oxford: Oxford University Press, 2010), S.V.: Beriberi.

43 George W. Bruyn and Charles M. Poser, *The History of Tropical Neurology: Nutritional Disorders* (Canton, MA: Science History Publications, 2003), 6.

44 See Kenneth J. Carpenter, *Beriberi, White Rice, and Vitamin B: A Disease, A Cause, and A Cure* (Berkeley: University of California Press, 2000).

45 A. J. Jefferson, "A case of pernicious beri-beri," *British Medical Journal*, 1950 (May 14, 1898): 1257.

46 The figures are extracted from respective annual reports of Colonial Surgeons in *Hong Kong Administrative Reports.*

47 C. A. Pekelharing and C. Winkler, *Beriberi: Researches Concerning Its Nature and Cause and the Means of Its Arrest,* translated by James Cantlie (Edinburgh: Young H Pentland, 1893).

48 Gibson, R. M. "Beriberi in Hong Kong, with Special Reference to the Records of the Alice Memorial and Nethersole Hospitals and with Notes on Two Years

Experience of the Disease." M.D. thesis, University of Edinburgh (1900). The catalogue at the HKU library does not specify that it was a higher degree thesis. According to Frank Shulman who has done extensive research in the bibliography of Hong Kong studies, it was a M.D. thesis.

In the original thesis, there was no abstract. Shulman has compiled the following abstract: "Gibson reported on medical developments in Hong Kong during two years of his residence in the colony. Utilizing the outpatient and inpatient registers for the years 1888–1889 inclusive of two hospitals that shared the same management and treated the local Chinese population free of charge, he studied a 'native disease' that was endemic in the tropical climate of Hong Kong and that reached an abnormal high of four hundred twenty-eight cases in 1899. He discussed the climatological causes of beriberi, the seasonal trends in its occurrence, its symptoms and diagnosis, the treatment of beriberi and related mortality rates, the characteristics of the children and adults who suffered from this disease, and the age of people when beriberi most commonly occurred. Gibson found that male coolies constituted the majority of the Chinese male beriberi patients. For purposes of illustration, he singled out nine cases that were based on his personal interaction with individuals who had beriberi at that time. Gibson's dissertation was submitted in the form of an unpaginated, handwritten text dated 'Hong Kong, 16th March 1900' that contained two photographs of hospital patients and reproduction of selected hospital records." See, *Doctoral Dissertations on Hong Kong 1900–1997* (Hong Kong: Hong Kong University Press, 2001), 277.

49 William Hunter and Wilfred Koch, *A Research into the Etiology of Beriberi; together with a report on an outbreak in the Po Leung Kuk* (Hong Kong, Hong Kong Government, 1906).
50 He wrote a long letter dated December 29, 1905 to explain his findings to the Governor of Hong Kong. See, ibid., 125–128.
51 Hunter and Koch, *A Research into the Etiology of Beriberi.*
52 Ibid., 148.
53 "The Far Eastern Association of Tropical Medicine," *British Medical Journal*, 2573 (April 23, 1910): 1000.
54 Government Notification No. 44, *The Hong Kong Government Gazette* (February 24, 1911): 59.
55 *Medical and Sanitary Reports for the Year 1914*, 22.
56 *Colonial Reports – Annual No. 282; Medical and Sanitary Reports for the Year 1914*; and Roger Bristow, *Land-use Planning in Hong Kong: History, Politics and Procedures* (Hong Kong: Oxford University Press, 1984), 35–37.

4   Disease, industrialization, and wartime destruction, 1920s–1945

During the interwar years, Hong Kong's fortunes continued to be closely intertwined with developments in China. The political and social turmoil as well as economic instability in China worsened despite the establishment of a new Republican government under Chiang Kai-shek in Nanjing in 1928. Chiang, in fact, not only had to deal with the continued challenge from the communists but also the expanding intrusion of Japan that, by the early 1930s, had become entrenched in China's northeastern provinces. On July 7, 1937, Japan began a full-scale invasion of China and quickly succeeded in controlling most of the eastern part of the country. These tumultuous developments created unprecedented social upheaval that resulted in large-scale population migrations inside China as well as the movement of hundreds of thousands of migrants and subsequently refugees into Hong Kong. While these newcomers brought capital as well as skilled and unskilled labor to the colony, their arrival also contributed to major problems of housing and public health. Britain downplayed the possibility of Japan invading Hong Kong or Singapore, stressing that both countries had been on good terms as allies since 1902.[1] The Japanese, however, did not spare Hong Kong. Japanese battalions moved near the border on December 4, 1941, and invasion of the colony began in the early morning hours of December 8. On Christmas Eve, Hong Kong Governor Mark Young surrendered, and the Japanese occupation of Hong Kong, which lasted until August 1945, began.[2] Wartime destruction was severe. More than a million people fled Hong Kong and those who stayed behind lived in fear and misery. The Japanese occupation was remembered by many as the darkest chapter in Hong Kong's history.

Industrialization and workers' conditions before the Japanese occupation

The 1920s and 1930s saw the continued shift of Hong Kong's economy from entrepot trade to manufacturing. While the influx of capital and refugees that provided both skilled and unskilled labor from China had facilitated this move, changes in the international economy also forced Hong Kong to adjust to new realities. Hong Kong's entrepot trade was badly hit by the severe worldwide economic depression in the late 1920s and early 1930s. Britain and its colonies devised a tariff system at the Imperial Economic Conference at Ottawa in 1932 that would create a zone of lower tariffs for goods within the British Empire. This so-called "imperial preference" therefore encouraged the development of industries in Hong Kong manufacturing goods for markets within the Empire.[3] At the same time, the emergence of economic nationalism in China led to a movement among many Chinese to promote the purchase of Chinese products while boycotting foreign goods.[4] Products from Chinese manufacturers in Hong Kong would therefore be preferred over foreign products in the China market.

Industrial activities expanded rapidly and the number of factories and workshops rose from around 200 in 1920 to 403 in 1933 and to 829 in 1938.[5] Ngo Tak Wing points out that the number of workers engaged in manufacturing accounted for "one quarter of the working population and one-seventh of the total population," as revealed in the 1931 census.[6] Investors in the manufacturing sector were mostly Chinese businessmen who focused mainly on light industries, with products such as cigars, tobacco, preserved fruits, and some household gadgets. In 1920, the amount of their investment amounted to HK$17.5 million. British investments, usually on a larger scale, were in heavy industries such as shipbuilding and repairing, and totalled around HK$50 million for the same year. By 1935, another survey revealed that Chinese investments in manufacturing had already exceeded HK$51 million. Ngo, however, argued that it was "a gross underestimation," pointing out that "many more industries had been set up, the larger ones included knitting and weaving, medicines and perfumery, printing and stationery, and rubber canvas shoes."[7] Some large factories such as Fung Keong Rubber Factory (founded in 1920), and Sam Hsing Weaving Factory (founded in 1929), might employ more than 2,000 workers. As for the value of exports, it could exceed HK$90 million annually between 1939 and 1940 – being "one-sixth of the value of Hong Kong's total export and re-export trade (HK$512 million) in 1938."[8] The Sino-Japanese War and tensions caused by the escalating military situation in different parts of the British Empire helped to generate strong demands for a wide range of products, from consumer goods to war materials and supplies such as electric hand-torches, dry batteries, rubber boots and shoes, gas masks, metal helmets, spades, uniforms, water-bottles, and portable military transmitting and receiving sets.[9] Based on the number of workers employed, the top five industries in Hong Kong in 1938 were: shipyards (10,426 workers), knitting factories (6,745 workers), spinning and weaving factories (6,151 workers), metal wares (3,926 workers), and rubber factories (2,019 workers).[10] Of the top five industries, with the exception of shipyards, female workers outnumbered male workers. A recent study shows that the ship-building capacity in Hong Kong had become a major one in Asian history – 10 major ships being made – contributing significantly to the Allied war efforts.[11] A government report of 1939 pointed out that "an outstanding feature [of the manufacturing industry] was the construction by local shipyards of the two largest ships ever built in the Colony.... Skilled labour was in demand principally in the shipyards and there was also a steady demand for both skilled and unskilled labour by military authorities."[12]

The rise of a nascent labor movement and the welfare of the workers, including health care, safety and working conditions, had emerged as significant social issues confronting the government since the 1920s. The emergence of "workers' collective consciousness" in Hong Kong could be attributed to political developments in South China. The Hong Kong Seamen's Strike in 1922 and the Guangdong Hong Kong General Strikes in 1925–1926 were good examples of the impact the bourgeoning labor movement in China had on Hong Kong's growing industrial proletariat.[13] As David Faure points out, "the political developments in China [in the 1920s] were fast creating the ideology of the working class."[14]

Labor affairs fell within the ambit of the Secretary for Chinese Affairs, and since the 1920s, the government had become concerned with the developing labor union movement, especially the potential of communist involvement. For example, a labor strike in 1928 at a rubber factory led the government to conclude that "the whole affair had been deliberately organized by two women Communists."[15] In November 1930, another strike of 600 female workers at a tobacco company was apparently caused by communist agitators.[16] In addition to being vigilant of communist activities, the government tried to forestall labor troubles by paying more attention to the wellbeing of the workers.

It should also be noted that the call by some missionaries to deal with the problem of child labor had already led to a series of public debates in London and Hong Kong that finally resulted in the enactment of the first legislation dealing with employment of children in industries in 1922.[17] But from the late 1920s to the 1930s, the government passed a number of legislations directed at the health and wellbeing of the workers. Ordinances to prevent industrial accidents were passed and revised during that period, with the intention of ensuring better protection of women and young workers and occupational safety. Moreover, child and women workers as well as young workers were forbidden to work in dangerous industries, and during night-shifts between late evening and early morning. Attempts were also made to improve health and industrial safety. For example, the government investigated potential mercury or other forms of poisoning of workers at the white lead and vermilion factories, and considered measures that could "be taken to minimise the risk from such industrial diseases."[18] Under the ambit of the Urban Council in 1938, Henry R. Butters, who had a deep knowledge of Hong Kong affairs, served as the Labor Officer,[19] and he completed a comprehensive study entitled *Report on Labour and Labour Conditions in Hong Kong*, a first of its kind in Hong Kong's labor history. He argued that the mere expression of support for labor was not enough. He proposed the expansion of labor welfare legislations to include a variety of health issues related to workers. For example, he wanted to put "occupational diseases in the proposed Workmen's Compensation Ordinance." Apart from occupational diseases (that included accidents),

Butters was aware of the prevalence of tuberculosis among the working poor, a disease attributable to their deplorable working and living conditions. Indeed, working conditions varied greatly, but most small industrial and sub-contractor workshops were "little better than urban slums where few or no amenities are provided for the workers."[20] Butters also pointed to the serious problem of opium or heroin addiction among the workers.[21] But the outbreak of the Sino-Japanese War and escalating military tensions in Asia precluded the possibility of translating his report into policy initiatives.

Demographic changes and housing

For most of the early twentieth century, the population of Hong Kong increased at a rapid pace. It was a result of the huge influx of Chinese migrants that, as noted, had contributed to Hong Kong's industrialization as well as to aggravating problems of housing and public health. The population figures of Hong Kong clearly illustrated the scope of growth: 585,090 in 1921, 849,750 in 1931, and 1,071,893 in 1940.[22] The figure in 1940 excluded the number of refugees, which was believed to be around 750,000. In other words, on the eve of the Japanese occupation of Hong Kong, the total population was 1.82 million. A significant feature was the changing distribution of the population as more and more people were moving to Kowloon since the City of Victoria had become overcrowded. The population in Kowloon jumped from 67,497 in 1911 to 123,448 in 1921, and from 270,940 in 1931 to 406,081 in 1940.[23] Such a shift was a result of the government's policy in developing Kowloon to enable population dispersal.[24] By 1932, 32 percent of the colony's population lived in Kowloon, and the percentage increased to 38 percent in 1940. As noted in the last chapter, the government had to expand public health services and medical services into the newly populated areas. Another important feature of the population was the changing ratio between males and females over these years. Specifically, the numbers of males per 100 females over these years dropped from 181 in 1911 to 135 in 1940.[25] The continued growth of the economy, especially the expansion of manufacturing industries offered more job opportunities for women workers who were needed in the bourgeoning industrial sector.

Not surprisingly, the ever-increasing population imposed a tremendous burden on existing housing that was already over-crowded, especially within the City of Victoria. The density had exceeded 1,200 people per acre in the mid-1920s and slightly decreased to approximately 1,000 people per acre by the early 1930s. Newly reclaimed areas were available for development, and Kowloon as well as New Kowloon, both of which had a density of around 300 people per acre, had become popular choices for relocation. One contemporary account indicated that in the City of Victoria, people lived in "tiers of bunks placed against the walls." Some people lived in cubicles as small as eight feet by eight feet with a height of six feet, and these were "more or less permanent homes of the people."

Throughout the 1930s, government health officials had constantly noted the critical relationship between public health and housing conditions. For example, one government director of medical services rightly pointed out that "the maintenance of a satisfactory standard of sanitation under such conditions is a most difficult problem and one which cannot be solved without the willing co-operation of the people. One thing is certain, so long as buildings are over-crowded and insanitary, no amount of external sanitation will give immunity from disease."[26] In 1935, the government formed a Housing Commission to investigate the problems of housing, and its report was released three years later. Governor Geoffrey Northcote supported a systematic approach to town planning and secured the support of the Finance Secretary to make available funding for the purpose from the Exchange Fund. But the unstable conditions caused by the Japanese invasion of China prevented the introduction of more vigorous and systematic town planning.[27] Conditions continued to deteriorate. Writing in April 1939, Butters in his report remarked that "a flat in normal times may have as many as twenty five adults stowed away in cubicles, bed spaces and cocklofts: and the population is at present [after the fall of Guangzhou in 1938] swollen with an addition of twenty five to fifty per cent, accommodated in existing houses."[28]

Diseases and public health

From the 1920s to the early 1940s, Hong Kong's economic expansion, and its ability to respond to changing regional and global markets in manufacturing goods, had been made possible, to a significant extent, by a fast-growing labor force composed of long-time residents as well as new migrants. Yet, the success was accompanied by the exacerbation of public health issues associated with the problem of unsanitary and congested housing conditions and deplorable working conditions in both big and small manufacturing industries.

Of the most prevalent diseases, respiratory diseases and pulmonary tuberculosis ranked first and second in the list of causes of death throughout these years. During the 1920s, the largest number of deaths caused by respiratory diseases, a total of 4,863, occurred in 1922, while a high of 4,411 pulmonary tuberculosis deaths was recorded in 1928. In the 1930s, the year with the highest mortality for both diseases was 1937, 10,380 for respiratory diseases and 3,061 for pulmonary tuberculosis.[29] Dr. Li Shu-fan, the superintendent of Hong Kong Sanatorium and Hospital (commonly known as Yeung Wo among the Chinese) noted that during the early 1920s, about 40 percent inpatients had tuberculosis. Li himself suffered from the ailment. In fact, he developed a new surgical procedure to treat the disease.[30]

As we have seen, except for public health education and anti-spitting propaganda, the government did not have a comprehensive and systematic approach to deal with these diseases. Government reports, while paying lip service to the need to act, inevitably singled out the root cause of the problem: poor housing conditions and poverty. One medical report, for example, stated that "the overcrowded houses, the expectorating habits of the people, and poverty furnish sufficient explanation for the prevalence of respiratory problems."[31] But the government was not about to provide massive welfare support to the population to lift them out of poverty. This position was expressed clearly in the Housing Committee report in 1938: "overcrowding arises almost entirely from poverty which in Hong Kong is so dire that many families cannot afford any rent at all...Poverty itself is the result of an economic system over which Government has little or no control."[32] Local voluntary organizations tried to provide some aid to alleviate the problem. Dr. Selwyn-Clarke, a newly appointed Director of Medical and Sanitary Services in 1937 founded the Anti-Tuberculosis Association with the assistance of several prominent local leaders. The association raised funds to support research and treatment of tuberculosis and promote health education and prevention. It also advocated pay raises for workers so that they would not go hungry and become more vulnerable if infected.[33]

The government, on the other hand, adopted a more systematic approach in its anti-malaria activities. Between 1920 and 1937, the average annual mortality rate of malaria was 489, but the major parts of urban Hong Kong and Kowloon fared much better than the suburbs and rural parts of the New Territories where some areas remained malarious.[34] In 1928, David Given, Naval Health Officer at Singapore criticized the Hong Kong government's inaction in malaria research. The government hired a malariologist, Dr. R.B. Jackson, and founded the Malaria Bureau in 1930 to conduct research in the epidemiology and control of malaria. The Bureau's work provided useful data for understanding the transmission of malaria in Hong Kong and the New Territories.[35] In major urban areas of Hong Kong and Kowloon, a drainage system was installed as a part of the anti-malaria infrastructure.[36] The government also reported that the construction of such major projects in the New Territories as the Shing Mun Dam and the Royal Air Force aerodrome was free from malaria problems.[37]

Impact of the Sino-Japanese War: refugees and health, 1938–1941

A pressing public health issue in Hong Kong since 1938 was the arrival of huge numbers of refugees fleeing the war-torn regions in nearby provinces. Between 1938 and 1939, 261,600 reached Hong Kong by railway and 327,833 by steamship.[38] The figures did not include refugees who reached Hong Kong by other unregistered vehicles or on foot. For example, on February 21, 1939, Japanese military operations in a nearby region drove out 50,000 refugees who walked miles to Hong Kong. In June 1939, the Hong Kong government estimated that the population was in the range of 1.8 to 2.2 million,[39] with an estimated 700,000 refugees.[40]

With an eye to social stability and public health, the government prioritized the refugee problem in its public policy. It opened three urban camps and five rural camps as well as utilized idle railway cars to shelter the refugees. These provisions were not enough, however, and there was great demand for short-term tenancy. It was estimated that 60 people, on average, shared an apartment. Rent was expensive and poor ventilation and unhygienic conditions in overcrowded tenements were of grave concern. To prevent the spread of diseases, in 1939, the government administered altogether 320,748 anti-cholera inoculations and 1,392,860 smallpox vaccinations. It made use of graphic posters to promote personal hygiene and appropriate preventive measures.[41]

Another urgent issue was food. Price for foodstuffs went up because the increase in demand far exceeded that of supply. Widespread malnutrition and deficiency diseases, such as beriberi, not to mention the potential of starvation, could be sources of social instability. The number of beriberi patients indeed increased over these years, from 563 in 1935 to 745 in 1936; although the numbers dropped slightly from 2,673 in 1937 to 2,061 in 1938.[42] The government adopted the extraordinary measure of price control over rice. It was made possible by the control over the rights of the import and sale of rice on the one hand, and through a sizable stock of rice as a price stabilizer to adjust the balance between supply and demand.[43] In 1939, the government delivered several hundred thousand of free meals at camps and welfare centres; the government also offered some assistance to voluntary organizations such as the Hong Kong Refugee and Social Welfare Council and Hong Kong Red Swastika Society for food aid to the poor. More importantly, the Hong Kong government established the Nutrition Research Committee in 1938, chaired by the Director of Medical and Sanitary Services. Through scientific study of meals provided at the refugee camps, the committee aimed at finding out "an economic but satisfactory dietary within the means of even the poorer class." They came up with a balanced diet that cost only 11.3 cents per day for those over seven years old and 8.2 cents for those up to seven years old.[44] The committee promoted the dietary formula through the radio and Chinese newspapers.

Socio-economic conditions under the Japanese occupation, 1941–1945

The Japanese occupation of Hong Kong saw the grave deterioration of socio-economic conditions. Despite propaganda promoting the "Greater East Asia Co-Prosperity Sphere," industry and commerce were at a standstill, and there was neither import of raw materials nor export of manufactured goods. There was a collapse of the basic social infrastructure and support: the Japanese took no action to rebuild damaged dwellings, to provide a sufficient supply of fuel and electricity and clean water, or to provide adequate protection of personal safety; moreover, the system of food rationing was ineffective and people had to depend upon the black market for food and drugs.[45] The Japanese were not about to take care of the huge population and the jobless were repatriated to their home countries. There were reports of extreme measures taken by the occupiers: "These [people being picked up from the streets] were towed out to sea and sunk or set on fire, charred bodies floating ashore afterwards," reported Dr Selwyn-Clarke.[46] Hong Kong's population was more than 1.7 million in 1941, and the figure dropped to 0.6 million when the Japanese surrendered in 1945.

Food and survival

Not surprisingly, food was a major problem during the occupation. Since rice was the staple food for most people, the government had, by the end of 1941, stockpiled up to 1,500,000,000 catties of rice that was thought to be enough to feed 1.7 million people for a period of up to eight months. Such a reserve could ensure an orderly market provided that import of rice could be maintained. Yet, the Japanese failed on both fronts: they seized all the rice depots and sold the rice based upon a system of rationing. The system collapsed in mid-1944 and the Japanese found it difficult to import rice from other parts of Southeast Asia especially since their control over Burma and the Philippines was falling apart in 1944. There was an astronomical rise in price:[47] in 1945, the price for one catty of rice was 270 Japanese military yen, or HK$1,080. In 1941, the price was only HK$0.2.[48] All kinds of foodstuffs were in serious shortage. People resorted to getting supplies and food, often of poor quality and suspicious origins, from the black market. The Japanese denied reports of cannibalism in Hong Kong, especially between 1944 and 1945.[49] When the British resumed control over Hong Kong after September 1945, their studies concluded that "over one third of the deaths" were attributed to either starvation or deficiency diseases.[50] Dr Li Shu-fan, the superintendent of the Yeung Wo Hospital, recorded the desperation of ordinary people: "it was pathetic to see poor people following a Japanese Army rice truck along the street in order to sweep up the few grains that might fall. Sometimes, starvelings would grab a bag from the truck, but they were invariably shot down."[51] Hong Kong Catholic Church Bishop Henry Valtoria chronicled the deadly consequences of the occupation as follows, "month after month, every day 300–400 corpses were collected in the urban streets, sometimes even more, reaching up to 721 one day, who died of hunger, exhaustion, or disease, to a total number of 50,000."[52]

Diseases, sanitation, and health

With Japan's occupation of Hong Kong, health conditions in the city deteriorated rapidly. According to Dr Li Shu-fan, "malignant malaria, cholera and other diseases were breaking out." It was due to "stagnant pools of water, fifthly tin cans, broken vessels and cesspools – all these, everywhere, were excellent breeding places for mosquitoes."[53] In fact, it was only the beginning of a catastrophic collapse of the health infrastructure. Anti-malarial work came to a halt and mosquitoes were everywhere. Metal was so important that heaps of tin were to be collected only by authorized agents. For security reasons, Japanese troops barricaded many buildings, making it impossible for workers to enter to check and empty open containers, such as tins and cans, of still water. Even worse, the Japanese refused to provide oil to insulate air from water surface to prevent the hatching of mosquito eggs. Whatever preventive measures were introduced proved to be incomplete and ineffective.[54] Second, there were outbreaks of cholera that spread rapidly in the poor and unsanitary environment. The mortality of cholera cases as recorded in hospitals in 1942 and 1943 was 58 percent.[55] An anti-cholera inoculation campaign proved futile as the Bacteriological Institute did not get necessary support in its production of anti-cholera vaccine. The vaccines that the Japanese produced were unfortunately "heavily contaminated." Similarly, the anti-smallpox vaccine was ineffective and the public refused to be vaccinated because syringes and needles were repeatedly used without sterilization. "Many inflamed arms and abscesses were encountered following these mass infected inoculations," one eyewitness commented.[56] There was a surge in tuberculosis cases as a result of Japanese inaction. The Anti-Tuberculosis Association maintained an underground treatment program until 1944 when all of its funding dried up. For those tuberculosis patients suffering from starvation or malnutrition, their chances of survival were almost non-existent as the Japanese occupiers were not about to share valuable medical resources with them.[57]

Venereal diseases and injuries caused by rape committed by Japanese soldiers were rampant. According to Dr. Selwyn-Clarke, "the Japanese troops were not content with using common prostitutes but forced others to their will."[58] Dr Li Shu-fan opined that "the Japanese government and the so-called Japanese military code condoned rape with the tacit understanding that it was one of the rewards if not the right of the conqueror."[59] Furthermore, he pointed to the physical as well as mental damages suffered by rape victims:

> Since Chinese women are modest, only a small percentage of those who were raped appeared at hospitals to be treated for rape injuries. They felt so ashamed and disgraced that most of them would rather have died than to have had it known... At my hospital we treated rape victims ranging from the early teens to the sixties. I myself treated and tried to comfort women with their teeth bashed in, their noses broken, their bodies showing bayonet prods; wives so heavy with child that the assault has brought on miscarriage; and young, tender girls whose minds had been affected by the pain and horror of multiple rape.[60]

There was also a collapse of the sanitary infrastructure. In Dr. Selwyn-Clarke's report, he singled out areas of general measures for sanitation in public health, namely, night-soil disposal and refuse disposal; drainage and water supply; mortuaries and cemeteries; markets and slaughter houses; restaurants and eating houses; food shops and food factories. The foundations of the basic sanitary measures were destroyed and supervision and management of these activities were impaired as professional personnel were interned. Saving energy, the Japanese did not use trucks to collect refuse and did not supply electricity for toilet flushing. Night-soil collection was left entirely to guild members who charged a high fee. Drainage was silted, creating ideal breeding places for mosquitoes. Water was not chlorinated and the supply filter was not cleaned and maintained. Mortuary and cemetery projects came to a halt. Finally, there were no clear regulations governing the sanitary requirements, and workers in markets, slaughter houses, restaurants, food shops, and factories could be sources of contamination and diseases such as cholera and dysentery.[61]

Hospitals and medical care

The hospital system that was in place before the Japanese occupation also suffered after the Japanese took over. All except five hospitals were made available for the exclusive use by Japanese troops and medical equipment in hospitals and clinics were deployed to the newly installed healing stations and hospitals. Between 1942 and 1945, Hong Kong had become one of the major healing stations for wounded soldiers from other parts of the Japanese Empire since medical equipment in Hong Kong hospitals was generally of better quality. A recent study shows that there were altogether 48 shipments from Southeast Asia, each of which could consist of up to a thousand wounded soldiers being transferred to Hong Kong for cure and recovery. For the Japanese occupiers, the biggest hospital project was to convert Kowloon Hospital into "The Hong Kong Army Hospital" (*Honkon Rikugun Byōin*) with the capacity to care for a total of 2,000 patients. Nearby schools were designated as subsidiary healing stations to accommodate more patients. The constant inflow of wounded soldiers apparently affected the morale among some Japanese soldiers as there were reports of escapes made by both wounded and serving soldiers.[62]

In Kowloon, the only hospital available for civilian use was Kwong Wah Hospital. It was, however, depleted of staff and medical supplies. According to the oral account of a nurse working at the hospital during the Japanese occupation, the medical service delivered was of low quality because of insufficient supply of medicine and food. A prevalent disease in Hong Kong at that time was dysentery, and segregation of patients, in this case, in a temporary hut with a capacity to hold 200, was the common practice to prevent further spread of the disease. But it was always overcrowded and understaffed – only two nurses were on duty, while two patients shared a bed. Under extreme circumstances, the space underneath the bed had to be utilized for patients as well. Beriberi and serious ulceration on the tongue were also most common. But no thiamine could be given, and steamed eggs would be available while stocks lasted. Doctors and nurses were short of medicine, and they had to resort to other simple and basic remedies. The worst part was the loss of trust among people. There was always the fear of betrayal that made life difficult and unbearable.[63]

On the Hong Kong side, Hong Kong Sanatorium & Hospital was of special significance. The hospital was private and it was managed solely by Chinese practitioners of Western medicine. It had advanced medical equipment and facilities. Once war broke out between Hong Kong and Japan, it became a government unit and the Chinese surgeons and physicians in private practice nearby were enlisted to serve. Dr. Li Shu-fan transformed the hospital into a major surgical center with an expanded capacity to handle 300 cases.[64] The many causalities caused by bombardment and combat demanded immediate care and surgery. The hospital was positioned as a "causality clearing unit," meaning that the patients would be discharged as soon as signs of recovery were noted.[65] After the Japanese occupied Hong Kong, the hospital was allowed to continue with its own management since it was privately owned and managed by Chinese practitioners of Western medicine. Dr. Li Shu-fan, the hospital superintendent, however, had to negotiate with the Japanese commander for the protection of nurses, and for the supply of electricity at a reduced price, especially since the use of X-ray was vital in surgery.[66] The hospital remained a target of Japanese extortion of money and presents and it managed to survive with the sale in the black market of their reserve medical supplies. The Japanese did not trust Dr. Li, however, and he successfully escaped from Hong Kong on August 1, 1943.[67] The hospital barely survived the occupation, and Dr. Li resumed his work in the hospital after the occupation ended.[68]

The camps

Under the occupation, British officials and officers were put into the prisoners-of-war camp while Western civilians were locked up in the internment camp. The internees were given only a meager amount of food, and very limited medical care was actually delivered by the physicians, surgeons, and dentists in the camp. The medical care within the civilian camp at Stanley, for example, was dependent on a limited provision of drugs and medical apparatus, most of which were smuggled into the camp through feeble social networks that the internees had established and managed to maintain under such unfavorable conditions. For humanitarian reasons, a few Japanese officers tacitly allowed this to continue.[69] Many diseases were prevalent: these included dysentery, diarrhoea, typhoid, tuberculosis, typhus, malaria, and those caused by malnutrition.[70] The internees carried out anti-malaria measures, for example, eliminating still water sources, to prevent the breeding of mosquitoes. There were 682 malaria cases at the Stanley camp, but not one mortality. Such diseases or physical disorders as beriberi, anaemia, central blindness, and visual disorder caused by under-nourishment were common, and some died as a result of their ailments.[71] Dr. Selwyn-Clarke identified a substantial amount of thiamine that was locked up in the vaults of the Hong Kong and Shanghai Bank, and managed to smuggle it into the camp so that the spread of beriberi was better controlled.[72] Life in the Sham Shui Po Prisoner-of-War Camp was harsher. Not only was it much more crowded with nearly 5,000 internees, but the Japanese also demanded internees to preform hard labor while living on a meager amount of food and very limited provisions of medical care delivered by their fellow internees.[73]

The last two paragraphs in Selwyn-Clarke's report that was written on January 31, 1946 aptly summed up the devastation suffered by Hong Kong during the occupation; and, at the same time, revealed the sanguine hope apparently shared by some British leaders at that time of good relations with a "young China." But in a few years' time, the rise of the People's Republic of China would radically alter the geopolitical landscape in Asia. He wrote:

> The systematic starving of the bulk of the population over such an extended period – over three and a half years – is likely to exercise a serious effect on the health of the community for many years to come, including an increase in the incidence of, and deaths from, tuberculosis. Hundreds of dwellings were destroyed by bomb, shell and fire during hostilities in 1941 and as the result of aerial bombings, but thousands of dwellings and many valuable educational establishments (e.g., the University of Hong Kong, Kings and Queens Colleges etc.) were irreparably damaged by looters whose activities could have been stayed by the Japanese.
>
> General hygiene (including water purification plants) suffered marked deterioration during the occupation of the Colony by a race which claimed to possess a higher standard of hygiene than any other in the world. The community was deprived of most of its medical and health services, its chief hospitals being taken for Japanese troops, its maternal, child welfare and social hygiene clinics closed and vital preventive work against malaria neglected. There is, however, another side to an otherwise sorely depressing picture. The ruthless invaders have given the British an opportunity of providing to young China the sincerity of their belief in the policy of co-partnership in the reconstruction of a new and better Hong Kong.[74]

The story of reconstruction and recovery from the damages of the war will be discussed in the next chapter.

Notes

1 Philip Snow, *The Fall of Hong Kong: Britain, China and the Japanese Occupation* (New Haven: Yale University Press, 2003).
2 For details of the Japanese military actions that led to the fall of Hong Kong, see Kwong Chi Man and Tsoi Yiu Lun, *Eastern Fortress: A Military History of Hong Kong, 1840–1970* (Hong Kong: Hong Kong University Press, 2014), 167–224.
3 Norman Miners, "Industrial development in the colonial Empire and the Imperial Economic Conference at Ottawa 1932," *The Journal of Imperial and Commonwealth History*, 30:2 (May 2002): 53–76.
4 For the practice and ideology of boycotting of foreign goods in the Chinese market during the 1920s and 1930s, see Marie-Claire Bergère, *The Golden Age of the Chinese Bourgeoisie 1911–1937*. Trans. Janet Lloyd (Cambridge: Cambridge University Press, 1986), 251–71.
5 For a general discussion of the growth of industries and the increase of industrial worker population, see Faure, "The common people in Hong Kong history: their livelihood and aspirations until the 1930s," 28–36.

6 Ngo Tak-wing, "Industrial history and the artifice of laissez-faire colonialism." In Ngo ed., *Hong Kong's History: State and Society under Colonial Rule*, 123.

7 Ngo Tak-wing, "The East Asian Anomaly Revisited: The Politics of Laissez-faire in Hong Kong, 1945–1985" (Ph.D. Thesis, University of London, 1996), 78.

8 Ngo, "Industrial history and the artifice of laissez-faire colonialism," 125.

9 *The Hong Kong Administrative Report for the Year of 1938*, 32.

10 Ibid.

11 Kwong and Lun, *Eastern Fortress*, 151.

12 *The Hong Kong Administrative Report for the year of 1939*, 22.

13 Ming K. Chan, "Labour vs crown: aspects of society-state interactions in the Hong Kong labour movement before WWII." In Elizabeth Sinn ed., *Between East and West: Aspects of Social and Political Development in Hong Kong* (Hong Kong: Centre of Asian Studies, Hong Kong University, 1990), 132–146.

14 Faure, "The common people in Hong Kong history: their livelihood and aspirations until the 1930s," 31.

15 *The Hong Kong Administrative Report for the year of 1928*, 29.

16 *The Hong Kong Administrative Report for the year of 1930*, K 14–15.

17 Carl T. Smith, "The first child labour law in Hong Kong." In *A Sense of History: Studies in the Social and Urban History of Hong Kong* (Hong Kong: Hong Kong Educational Publishing Company, 1995), 213–239.

18 *The Hong Kong Administrative Report for the year of 1928*, 29.

19 For his postings in 1938, see *The Hong Kong Blue Book for the year of 1938,* J2, J7, and J49.

20 Faure, *A Documentary History of Hong Kong: Society*, 202.

21 Henry Robert Butters, *Report on Labour and Labour Conditions in Hong Kong* (No. 8 of 1939) in *Sessional Papers for the Year of 1939*, 153–55.

22 The figures are extracted from the *Hong Kong Blue Books* in 1911, 1921, 1931, and 1940.

23 For the figures in 1911 and 1921, see "Report of the Census of the Colony for 1921," No. 15 of *Sessional Paper for the Year of 1921*, 174. For figures from 1931 and 1940, See *Hong Kong Blue Book for the year of 1931* and *Hong Kong Blue Book for the year of 1940*.

24 The problem in housing also attracted attention in other parts of China. For example, O. M. Green, "The coming city of Kowloon: Hong Kong Government's housing and reclamation," *North China Herald* (December 29, 1923).

25 The figures for male and female population over these years are as follows: 289,752 males and 160,346 females in 1911, 351,580 males and 234,300 females in 1921, 487,835 males and 361,915 females in 1931, and 615,451 males and 456,442 females in 1940. These figures are extracted from the *Hong Kong Blue Books* in 1911, 1921, 1931, and 1940.

26 "Medical and Sanitary," *Administrative Report for the year of 1931*, M 10.

27 Gavin Ure, *Governors, Politics and the Colonial Office: Public Policy in Hong Kong, 1918–1958* (Hong Kong: Hong Kong University Press, 2012), 139.

28 H. R. Butters, "Report on Labour and Labour Conditions in Hong Kong" (No. 3 of *Sessional Paper of the Year of 1939)*, 150.

29 See the sections on vital statistics and public health in the respective years of *Hong Kong Administrative Reports*.

30 Li Shu-fan, *Hong Kong Surgeon* (New York: E. P. Dutton & Co., 1964), 66.

31 Almost identical wordings were found in the government administrative reports from 1931 to 1939. See the section "Public Health" in the respective reports.

32 Hong Kong Government, *Report of the Housing Commission 1935* (No. 12 of *Sessional Paper for the year of 1938*), 260.

33 See Jones, "British Colonial Health Policy, 1900–1940: Ceylon and the Asian Colonies," 154–159.

34 The average is calculated from figures published in the sections "Vital Statistics" and "Public Health" in the *Hong Kong Administrative Reports* from 1920 to 1937.

35 Yip, "Colonialism, Disease, and Public Health: Malaria in the History of Hong Kong," 21–22.

36 "Public Health," *Administrative Report for the Year of 1931*, 7.

37 A. R. Wellington, "Memorandum regarding changes in the public health organization of Hong Kong during the period 1929 to 1937" (No. 4 of *Sessional Papers for the Year 1937*), 109.

38 "Medical and Sanitary," Administrative Report of Hong Kong for the year of 1939, M4.

39 Ibid., M7.

40 *Hong Kong Blue Book for the Year of 1939*, N1; as well as, *Hong Kong Blue Book for the Year of 1940*, N1.

41 "Public Health," *Administrative Report of Hong Kong for the year of 1939*, 4.

42 The figures are extracted from the respective years of the sanitary report. The figure was not given in the 1939 report.

43 Zheng Hongtai (Victor Cheng) and Huang Shaolun (Wong Siu-lun), *Xianggang Miye Shi* [A History of Rice Trade in Hong Kong] (Hong Kong: Joint Publishing Co., 2005), 74–84. For a general history of the rice trade in the first half of the twentieth century, see David Faure, "The rice trade in Hong Kong before the Second World War." In Elizabeth Sinn ed., *Between East and West: Aspects of Social and Political Devlopment in Hong Kong*, 216–225.

44 "Medical and Sanitary," *Administrative Report of Hong Kong for the year of 1939*, M8.

45 For details, see G. B. Endacott, *Hong Kong Eclipse* (Hong Kong: Hong Kong University Press, 1978), 139–164.

46 Selwyn Selwyn-Clarke, *Footprints: The Memoirs of Sir Selwyn Selwyn-Clarke* (Hong Kong: Sino-American Publishing Company, 1975), 69.

47 Guan Lixiong (Kwan Lai Hung), *Rizhan shiqi de Xianggang* [*The Japanese occupation of Hong Kong*] (Hong Kong: Joint Publishing Company, 1993), 92–102.

48 Selwyn Selwyn-Clarke, *Report on the Medical and Health Conditions in Hong Kong for the Period 1ˢᵗ January 1942–31 August 1945* (London: HMSO, 1946), 4.

49 Xie Yongguang, *Sannian ling bage yue de kunan* [Hardship and sufferings under the Japanese occupation of Hong Kong], 2nd ed. (Hong Kong: Ming Pao Publishing Co., 1995), 130–136.

50 Selwyn-Clarke, *Report on the Medical and Health Conditions in Hong Kong*, 7.

51 Li, *Hong Kong Surgeon*, 161.

52 Sergio Ticozzi, *Historical Documents of the Hong Kong Catholic Church* (Hong Kong: Hong Kong Catholic Diocesan Archives, 1997), 162.

53 Li, *The Hong Kong Surgeon*, 103.

54 Selwyn-Clarke, *Report on the Medical and Health Conditions in Hong Kong*, 12.

55 Ibid., 8.

56 Ibid., 13.

57 Ibid., 7.

58 Ibid., 8.

59 Li, *Hong Kong Surgeon*, 111.

60 Ibid.,111.

61 Selwyn-Clarke, *Report on the Medical and Health Conditions in Hong Kong*, 8–11.

62 Kuang Zhiwen (Kwong Chi Man), *Chongguang zhilu: Riju Xianggang yu Taiping yang zhanzheng,1942–1945* [Road to Liberation: Hong Kong under Japanese occupation and the Pacific War 1942–1945] (Hong Kong: Cosmos, 2015), 278–279.

63 "An oral history of Zheng Xiaoying," in Liu Zhipeng and Zhou Jiajian ed., *Tun sheng ren yu: Ri zhi shi qi Xianggang ren de ji ti hui yi* [The Tests of Endurance and Sufferance: An oral history of Hong Kong people during the Japanese occupation] (Hong Kong: Zhonghua Bookstore, 2009), 191–209.

64 Li, *Hong Kong Surgeon*, 95.
65 Ibid., 105
66 Ibid., 137.
67 Ibid., 140–181.
68 *Yanghe Yiyuan Lishi, 1922–2012* [History of the Hong Kong Sanatorium & Hospital, 1922–2012] (Hong Kong: Hong Kong Sanatorium & Hospital, 2012), 29.
69 Selwyn-Clarke, *Footprints*, 69–76. The story of smuggling a dentist chair into the camp is an example, see 75–76.
70 Geoffrey C. Emerson, *Hong Kong Internment 1942–1945: Life in the Japanese Civilian Camp at Stanley.* Reprint edition (Hong Kong: Hong Kong University Press, 2009), 105.
71 Ibid.,106–114. Detailed reports about the health situation in the Stanley Camp are also available in Selwyn-Clarke, *Report on the Medical and Health Conditions in Hong Kong*, 19–37.
72 Selwyn-Clarke, *Footprints*,75.
73 Considerable numbers of faculty members and students were kept in the camps. They became sources of information about the lives in the camp. See, Cunich, *A History of the University of Hong Kong*, 410–11.
74 Selwyn-Clarke, *Report on the Medical and Health Conditions in Hong Kong*, 18.

5 Health, disease control, and postwar reconstruction, 1945–1960s

The British reasserted control over Hong Kong after Japan surrendered on August 14, 1945. Although Chiang Kai-shek and the Chinese Nationalist government had been expected to retake the British colony, yet under pressure from the U.S., Chiang reluctantly agreed to let the British take the surrender of the Japanese at Hong Kong.[1] Both Chiang and the Chinese Communists were preoccupied with consolidating their respective positions in China before the inevitable showdown that finally came in 1949 when Chiang was ousted from the mainland and relocated to Taiwan. With the emerging Cold War and the establishment of the PRC, the United States saw Hong Kong as a useful and strategic outpost to counter the rise of communism. Although the PRC insisted that the resolution of the status of Hong Kong was a domestic matter, yet it was not prepared in the immediate postwar period to act precipitously for fear of provoking international intervention; moreover, its involvement in the Korean conflict in 1950 prevented further action as far as Hong Kong was concerned.

On May 1, 1946, Sir Mark Young became the governor of Hong Kong and restored civil administration to the colony. The short military administration that preceded Young had succeeded in restoring some semblance of social and economic order damaged by the Japanese occupation. Britain's prestige had declined as a result of the war, and in the colony, there was increasing demand for reform. Moreover, from 1946 to 1949, industrial action taken by workers demanding higher wages broke out and there were also conflicts between pro- and anti-communist groups. Even British expatriates insisted that "reform was essential if Britain was to hold on to Hong Kong."[2] Some social relief measures were introduced, including food kitchens to provide free meals and public work projects to reduce unemployment. Moreover, Young eased some of the prewar residential restrictions imposed on the Chinese, and introduced a "localization" program designed to recruit more local people into government service.[3] He proposed introducing a municipal council with most of its members popularly elected. However, the Young Plan, as it was called, was shelved after he left office, and Hong Kong's colonial state structure remained basically the same until the 1980s.[4] The tenure of the new governor, Sir Alexander Grantham, was rather uneventful except for the riots in October 1956 when supporters of the Nationalist government in Taiwan attacked communist areas and sympathizers over a dispute involving the removal of some Nationalist flags on October 10, the anniversary of the 1911 Revolution and the founding of the Republic of China. The government took decisive action and the riots quickly died down. Despite this incident, Hong Kong under Grantham managed to maintain stable relations with China, Taiwan, and the US. Another important legacy of Grantham was his decision to develop housing programmes in an attempt to help resettle the huge influx of refugees after a disastrous fire in a squatter area in 1953. His successor, Sir Robert Black whose tenure lasted from 1958 to 1964, continued the policy of pro-business and minimal intervention on behalf of the needy. His obituary in *The Economist* on November 4, 1999, in fact described his tenure in Hong Kong as "a period of money-making bliss that it never quite recaptured."[5] Under Grantham, taxes were low and public expenditures were carefully monitored and circumscribed. It was during the period of economic growth from the second half of the 1950s to the early 1960s that Hong Kong moved aggressively against communicable diseases so as to ensure a healthy environment and labor force vital to Hong Kong's economic expansion.

Economic reconstruction

A major concern of the postwar administration was of course Hong Kong's economic recovery after the devastation suffered during the Japanese occupation. External trade had come to a standstill, and industrial activities had become negligible. Without a viable economy, the colony's very survival was at stake – not to mention the government's ability to provide social services, including education, public health, and medical care. With the establishment of the PRC in 1949 and its recognition by Britain, Hong Kong was able to continue its commercial activities and trade with China. The outbreak of the Korean War and the subsequent embargo imposed on trade with China severely affected Hong Kong's entrepot trade with China as well as with other countries. The business community recognized the need to make structural adjustments in the economy and began to revitalize the manufacturing sector. Fortunately, as in the 1920s and 1930s, the influx of capital, entrepreneurs, and industrialists from Shanghai, skilled labor, and refugees seeking work from the mainland after 1949 provided the requisite conditions for the colony not only to recover from wartime destruction, but also expand upon the industrial base during the 1950s and early 1960s. The refugees in fact constituted a pool of valuable cheap labor willing to work for low wages and played a vital role in Hong Kong's development of the postwar industrial economy. Moreover, thanks to the government's determination to maintain Hong Kong as a free port and trading center, as well as the low tax environment and controls on public spending, Hong Kong was able to accelerate its economic growth. The government also encouraged labor-intensive industrialization to generate new sources of revenue.[6] By the end of the 1950s, more than 170,000 people were employed in 4,541 factories, and 69.9 percent of the colony's exports were goods made in Hong Kong. By the early 1960s, such industries as textiles, garments, plastics, electronics, watches, and toys grew rapidly and the manufacturing sector continued to expand in the early 1970s.[7]

The refugee problem

At the war's end, many who had fled the colony returned, boosting the colony's population to about 1.8 million by 1948. The civil war in China and the victory of the Communists led to a rapid and huge influx of refugees from the mainland, and Hong Kong's population surged to an estimated 2.3 million by May 1950.[8] The colonial government had rationalized initially that when the situation in China stabilized, many of these newcomers would leave. When this did not happen, the question became one of how to accommodate this unprecedented influx of population, the majority of whom were destitute and in urgent need of relief. Those fortunate enough to have relatives or friends to shelter them in the already overcrowded prewar Chinese tenements actually helped to exacerbate the congested and unsanitary living conditions of the poor. Many of these tenements were subdivided into tiny cubicles for multiple families that lived in the squalid environment with poor ventilation – not surprisingly, tuberculosis was prevalent and remained one of the most serious public health problems.

Most of the refugees, however, crowded into squatter camps that began to mushroom in hillsides, and in and around the city. It has been estimated that between 1949 and 1956, the squatter population increased from 30,000 to 300,000. One of the last cadet officers of the colonial government described the government's policy this way: "I had to manage the screening of squatters cleared for development when all they were offered as resettlement was four pegs in the ground making a plot where they could build. Gradually a little government money was found to do some site formation, to provide stand-pipes, to pave paths, to do a good deal but not to provide housing."[9] In addition to the refugees, the squatter camps were also home to many indigenous poor, including long-term city residents who had been evicted from condemned buildings or from older houses being demolished for redevelopment. A tiny hut of 40 square feet, made of wood, metal sheets, or even cardboards, would house five to six people. The dense overcrowding and poor living conditions were exacerbated by the ways that some of the dwellings were put to use: small factories, shops, schools, and brothels were to be found within the settlements. Not surprisingly, in addition to the fire hazard, these camps, most of them without running water or sanitary facilities, would provide ideal breeding grounds for diseases.[10]

To reduce health risks and fire hazards, the government began in July 1951 a resettlement program to remove squatters to either "approved" areas (i.e., land that would be costly or difficult to develop for other purposes), or "tolerated" areas located away from urban centers. In the former, squatters could build semi-permanent brick or stucco cottages with their own funds or support from charitable organizations. On the other hand, squatters could build on "tolerated" areas, wooden huts more or less as they saw fit. Both areas would be supplied with communal water taps and toilets. The government made it clear that resettlement was necessary not only for public health reasons, but also for the maintenance of social order – not to mention that the land illegally occupied proved to be valuable for urban development. Problems involving inadequate funding support, or the remoteness of locations in the tolerated areas that made it difficult for people to travel to work, however, made it clear that alternative resettlement schemes would be needed.[11]

The event that precipitated a major initiative in housing policy for the refugees was the disastrous fire that consumed the Shek Kip Mei squatter area in northern Kowloon on the night of December 25, 1953. More than 50,000 were rendered homeless. The government finally decided on a housing policy that involved a pilot project to construct several permanent six-story buildings at the site; this project would eventually become the prototype for future resettlement housing.[12] In the second half of the 1950s, the resettlement estates were organized in typical back-to-back "H blocks" with tiny family units and communal sanitary facilities. By early 1964, 13 resettlement estates were built. The severity and lamentable state of the housing situation was revealed in the 1961 census in which the code plan for the classification of accommodations for residents included cocklofts, staircases, passages, hawker stalls, caves, tunnels, and sewers![13] Moreover, the government also began to look for sites in the New Territories for urban and industrial development, a process that resulted in the development of new towns in rural areas, a topic that will be discussed in detail in the next chapter.

Public health policy and priorities

As noted, since the government believed at first that many of the refugees would leave Hong Kong when conditions in China improved, it was not prepared to invest much resources to provide needed social services for fear that such measures would actually attract more refugees. The relocation of the refugees into tolerated and approved areas was designed to reduce health and fire risks. Some minimal public health and sanitary measures were also implemented: for example, inoculation against cholera, vaccination, and the liberal use of insecticide on soiled areas. Moreover, in some camps, latrines were set up by the Urban Council that was responsible for environmental sanitation, and education in trash disposal was arranged.[14]

As in the past, the government's policy had been to rely heavily on voluntary and charitable organizations to provide resettlement assistance and some urgently needed social services to the refugees and the poor. The Tung Wah Group of Hospitals, for example, helped to mediate between some of the refugees and the government, and also provided assistance during the reset-tlement process.[15] Religious agencies such as the National Catholic Welfare

Conference and the World Council of Churches distributed relief materials and basic necessities, although on a temporary basis. UNESCO also distributed food and clothing to the refugees, in addition to maintaining clinics for the sick. After investigating the refugee situation in Hong Kong, Edvard Hambro, Chief of the Hong Kong Refugee Survey Mission sent by the UN High Commissioner for Refugees, concluded that "for all practical purposes the needs [of the refugees] are unlimited."[16] In December 1958, after the passage of the World Refugee Year Resolution in the UN General Assembly, aid was sent to refugees in Hong Kong. The funds collected during the refugee year were channeled into social services run by the government: for example, construction of schools and vocational training centers, libraries, and tuberculosis sanatoriums.[17]

The government's public health concerns were of course not confined to the refugees. The total population of Hong Kong grew to 1.8 million in 1948, from a low of about 600,000 in 1945. By mid-1950, the population stood at more than 2.2 million, and the census of 1961 revealed a total of about 3.1 million people.[18] Infant mortality rate improved slightly from 102.3 in 1947 to 99.6 per thousand live births in 1950, and it further dropped to 66.4 per thousand live births in 1955. These figures reflected the general amelioration of living conditions as well as the increase in the actual number of births registered. The general death rate, for 1950, on the other hand, was a rather low 8.2 per 1,000 of population, and it remained the same in 1955. According to the government, the low rates were likely a result of the absence of major epidemics or severe nutritional disorders, although it also pointed out that the rates were calculated using only estimated populations.[19]

During the immediate postwar period, the government was determined to promote economic growth through reestablishing Hong Kong's position as a premier trading center and international port. Consequently, it concentrated resources on the control of communicable diseases that threatened the development of a healthy labor force as well as invited international sanctions if Hong Kong became an infected port. Despite the heavy demand for social services posed by the influx of refugees, the government did not waver in its efforts to develop quarantine and epidemiological services dealing with communicable diseases. Tuberculosis and smallpox were especially targeted because of overcrowding, poor housing, exiguous water supplies, and general unsanitary conditions created the ideal environment for epidemics to occur. Moreover, to cut down the high maternal and infant mortality and apparently to ensure a healthy work force in the future, emphasis was placed on developing a maternity and child health service based on special clinics. This concentration of resources on prevention and disease control proved to be successful, and by the second half of the 1960s, Hong Kong's disease profile was transformed from one dominated by communicable diseases to one in which chronic diseases became increasingly important. This policy, however, prioritized prevention and disease control, rather than curative medical care. Certainly, the government did introduce medical services, but it clearly depended to a significant extent on the initiatives and activities of voluntary, charitable, and religious organizations as far as medical services were concerned.[20]

Disease prevention and control

The rapid increase in population and overcrowded and poor living conditions for the majority of the population had been recognized as the main causes of the prevalence of such diseases as tuberculosis, diphtheria, measles, pneumonia, gastro-enteritis, and the enteric fevers. In his 1955–1956 report, the medical director called these diseases either "diseases of congestion" or "diseases associated with dirt."[21] In his report on tuberculosis in 1950, A. S. Moodie, the government tuberculosis specialist, insisted that "the most obvious and urgent measure" to control the spread of tuberculosis "is to reduce the density of the population either by a reduction in the overall population, or by a very substantial increase in the housing accommodation."[22] In that year, tuberculosis accounted for 17.7 percent of the deaths from all causes, and was the most important single disease in the list of causes of death. What was particularly worrisome was the dramatic jump in tuberculosis mortality for the under-five-year age group – an increase of 41 percent from 1949 – clearly a result of gross overcrowding in homes, according to Moodie.[23] By 1953, tuberculosis had reached "almost epidemic proportions with a very high infection rate in early life, a high morbidity and mortality under five years of age, and almost universal infection in adults."[24]

Several preventive measures against tuberculosis were implemented. The most important was BCG vaccination that became widely used only after World War II. Other measures included X-ray surveys, contact examinations, and health education and social assistance. From 1952–1955, a BCG vaccination campaign that targeted newborns as well as school entrants who were aged about seven years was carried out with assistance from WHO and UNICEF. X-ray surveys for selected groups, including government employees, school teachers, and prisoners, were implemented because there were not enough resources and facilities to take care of the general population. To prevent the spread of infection, contacts of known cases of tuberculosis were examined and evaluated. Those under eight years old would be given a tuberculin test, and if found negative, would receive BCG vaccination. For every diagnosed case, almoners and tuberculosis visitors would follow up with interviews to determine the home environment and conditions. Financial assistance was available for the needy to undergo treatment. Specific health education for families during home visits or general health education for the public was carried out.[25] The BCG campaign proved to be extremely effective and the infant mortality rate from tuberculosis declined from 3.5 per 1000 live births in 1952 to virtually nil in 1971.[26] For those requiring treatment, the government operated several chest clinics which referred serious cases for hospital care. Significantly, the government offered free medical care to all needy tuberculosis patients.[27]

In the anti-tuberculosis efforts, the government was assisted by the Hong Kong Anti-Tuberculosis Association, a private philanthropic organization founded in October 1948. It established the Ruttonjee Sanatorium, named after its founder, and also maintained two other institutions for the treatment of tuberculosis; all three institutions received some form of government support. Moreover, the Association operated a BCG clinic and worked with the government in the BCG vaccination campaign. The Tung Wah Group of Hospitals reserved a block of beds for tuberculosis patients and participated in the BCG vaccination campaign, especially for babies born in the hospitals. Once again, the cooperation of the Hong Kong Anti-Tuberculosis Association and the government provided a good example of the mixed local voluntarism-government intervention in social amelioration that characterized the government's approach to providing social services.[28] These anti-tuberculosis efforts, both preventive and curative, proved to be successful as the percentage of deaths from the disease in relations to total deaths in the population fell from about 20 percent to 2 percent in the period from 1951 to 1977.[29]

The destruction of the public health infrastructure during the Japanese occupation had resulted in a major surge in malaria morbidity and mortality. In 1946, there were 2,400 cases with 765 deaths. In fact, the immediate postwar years witnessed an average of 1,100 cases per year with annual deaths ranging from 116 to 765, although mortality gradually declined in the 1950s.[30] The Malaria Bureau which was established in 1930, was reconstituted after the war and continued its research and anti-malaria activities. Anti-malaria activities in the postwar years became part of the concerted and broadly based efforts promoted by the government to control communicable diseases.

The availability of DDT and newly developed insecticides added to the arsenal that the Malaria Bureau could use in its anti-malaria programs. Residual spraying by DDT was carried out mostly in locations in the New Territories, including government quarters, and perimeter villages surrounding army camps.[31] Hong Kong, however, did not participate in the global malaria eradication campaign using DDT initiated by WHO. The government did try aerial spraying in 1946 but concluded that the blanket residual spraying of DDT was not necessary in Hong Kong and that the malaria control measures, especially the anti-larval program, that were in place would be more appropriate and economical.[32] Another important consideration was that as Hong Kong became urbanized, the build-up areas reduced the breeding grounds for mosquitoes. In the urban areas, the government continued the anti-vector program of proper drainage, sanitation improvements, and the elimination of potential breeding grounds for mosquitoes. It was in the New Territories, however, where infections remained high, and there was still no overall control program as late as 1960. The scattered population and the widespread wet cultivation made it difficult to implement such a program. In particular, the large majority of cases were found in Sai Kung, a small town on the east coast.[33] The situation would change during the second half of the 1960s as new towns were developed in the New Territories, resulting in increased urbanization of the formerly largely rural areas.

Thanks to the prewar vaccination campaign, smallpox, a notifiable disease subject to international quarantine, had declined in importance. With the influx of refugees, the government continued the vigorous vaccination campaign each winter, focusing in the first place on the squatter areas. During the immediate postwar years, between 1 and 1.5 million vaccinations had been carried out. From 1948 to 1951, only a total of 20 cases were notified. No cases were reported in 1954 and 1955, and there were no deaths from the disease.[34] In 1958, the WHO initiated a worldwide smallpox eradication program that had the ultimate objective of eradication in four or five years. From 1959 to 1966, countrywide elimination was achieved in countries in Asia, Africa, and the Americas. In October 1977, the last naturally transmitted case of smallpox occurred in Mogadishu, Somalia.[35] The WHO began certifying eradication of the disease from countries in 1973; and in July 1979, Hong Kong was certified to be smallpox free.

As in the case of controlling smallpox, immunization was the key in the government's attempt to combat cholera. Since cholera is a disease of poor environmental hygiene and sanitation, the deplorable living conditions in squatter camps and old tenements, exacerbated by the chronic shortage of water, provided ideal conditions for potential contamination of food and water that caused the disease. After the war, the Urban Council was responsible for the inspection of cleanliness of buildings and markets, as well as food and meat inspection to ensure the absence of contamination. But it was the vigorous inoculation campaign against cholera that helped to reduce or eliminate the possibility of outbreaks. The last case of cholera was reported in 1947. In 1950 alone, more than 600,000 cholera inoculations were carried out. As in the case of smallpox, the squatter areas were targeted first before other areas of the community. Firms and factories with a staff of 50 or over also received special priority in the inoculation campaign, although members of the public could get free inoculations at all government hospitals and clinics.[36] However, in mid-August 1961, a serious epidemic of a new subtype of cholera called cholera El Tor broke out in Hong Kong. This epidemic and the government's attempts to control the outbreak marked an important step in the development of public health measures to combat and control infectious diseases and will be discussed in detail in the next chapter.

Disease prevention and control: public health services

To carry out disease prevention and control programs, the government's Medical Department was divided into two divisions: the Health Division was responsible for the formulation and implementation of preventive measures, while the Medical Division took charge of the curative and investigative aspects of medical care. The Health Division's duties were extremely broad as it dealt not only with the general hygiene and sanitation of the city, but also specialized functions such as coordinating immunization campaigns, as well as anti-tuberculosis and anti-malaria activities. Moreover, it oversaw the Social Hygiene Service for the control and treatment of venereal diseases, the Maternal and Child Health Service, School Health Service, and the Port Health Service. By the mid-1950s, an Industrial Health Service was established to deal with health issues associated with the burgeoning manufacturing economy. In 1960, the Public Health and Urban Services Ordinance centralized functions concerned with the environmental services in the city, including the New Territories, and the Medical and Health Department had a closer working relationship with the Urban Council which was responsible for environmental sanitation.[37]

The Urban Council, re-constituted after the war, continued to be the primary agency responsible for the control of communicable diseases through improved environment sanitation, food hygiene, and vector control. The Council was also involved in the clearing of squatters and their resettlement. Over the years, the scope of the Urban Council's activities expanded to include recreational venues and activities and art and cultural development. On the other hand, medical and health officers in the urban areas coordinated all epidemiological measures to control the transmission of infectious disease except for tuberculosis, venereal disease, and malaria which were under direct control of specialized branches of the Department. As for the New Territories with its gradual urbanization and ever growing population, the responsibility for the extension of environmental health services remained with the Medical and Health Department. Residents were encouraged and educated to maintain environmental sanitation in their community.[38]

To ensure a healthy population in the future, the government paid a lot of attention to maternity and child welfare. In the immediate postwar period, maternity and child welfare centers were set up to provide pre- and post-natal counselling. The population served by these centers, however, remained limited as tight fiscal policy prevented the setting up of more centers. Investigation of the home environment and feeding habits of infants were carried out; in 1950, one report vividly described the unhealthy living conditions that most infants and mothers had to endure. The report pointed out that

> most of these mothers are living in poor and overcrowded conditions w[h]ere a whole family of five or six may have only a curtained-off cubicle enclosing an area of perhaps no more than 64 square feet, with no window, and there may be as many as five or six of these cubicles on one tenement floor opening onto the outside air at one end only...and... cooking facilities are limited and communal to the whole floor and that the water supply is cut off for long periods during the day and most of the night.

These conditions, according to the report, were the "root cause of the very high incidence of enteritis of infants, and possibly of broncho-pneumonia."[39]

As we have seen, overcrowded housing had already been a problem in the prewar period, and the government's housing policy in the immediate postwar years and the ever-increasing population precluded any large-scale and fundamental improvements in living conditions for the poor.

During the 1950s, the number of maternal and infant centers expanded, and their functions continued to focus on health education and the prevention of disease. If disease was detected, the mother or child would be referred to receive appropriate medical care. Immunizations against diphtheria, whooping cough, and tetanus were given, and smallpox vaccination was given where necessary; all children were tested for tuberculosis and those with a negative reaction received BCG vaccination. The services were provided free of charge and selected families of the lowest income groups enjoyed free supplementary meals at the centers. Again, international organizations, in this case UNICEF, offered skimmed milk powder and soap to the centers, while WHO also assisted the development of the program from 1954 to 1956. Local voluntary associations such as the *kaifongs* actively promoted health education related to maternal and infant welfare and in 1960 organized a three-month drive to educate the community in improvements in standards of maternal and child health.[40]

The School Health Service targeting students had similar objectives as the general sanitation improvement and disease prevention programs. Schools were periodically inspected to ensure cleanliness, proper ventilation, and sanitary arrangements. Health education, an essential part of the service, provided students, parents, and teachers with the latest information on preventive activities and disease control. The service also carried out immunization against diphtheria, cholera, and smallpox as well as BCG vaccination if necessary. Since the government did not have the funds nor facilities to provide curative care to all school students, it provided curative services only to a limited number of voluntary participants in a fee-paying scheme. Because of the overwhelming number of applicants, no new ones were accepted after 1955.[41] Later, in 1964, a new School Medical Service would be inaugurated.

The bourgeoning manufacturing sector of the economy necessitated special attention to the health hazards and environmental hygiene of the working environment as well as health and safety of the workers in order to sustain the valuable workforce. The Industrial Health Section of the Labor Department was staffed by officers seconded from the Medical and Health Department. It conducted field surveys of various industrial environments and working conditions; workers most likely exposed to health risks and toxins in their work were monitored through regular blood and urine examinations in the Industrial Hygiene Laboratory opened in the mid-1960s. Voluntary associations again took part in the promotion of safety in the work place, and the St. John's Ambulance Association conducted training classes in first aid for industries.[42] All these programs proved to be valuable to the protection of Hong Kong's labor force; however, a large number of the workers were still unable to benefit from them, either because of the limited scope of the programs, or because many of the working poor were sub-contractors who had turned their homes into small workshops. Conditions in these workshops were unsanitary and unhealthy, while safely standards were often non-existent. The problems of these workshops would intensify in the 1970s.

Since Hong Kong was a busy international port, it was vulnerable to imported diseases. Moreover, its proximity to southern China and other Asian cities where some infectious diseases such as malaria were endemic made it imperative that Hong Kong remained vigilant in monitoring incoming traffic, whether by sea, air, or land. The responsibility of the Port Health Administration was therefore to ensure that no quarantinable infectious diseases entered the city. It had marine quarantine anchorages to inspect incoming ships. To destroy rats and other pests, a fumigation service for ships and outgoing cargo was provided. The Port Health Administration was also responsible for controlling and inspecting traffic at the airport and the border crossing. For planes landing from infected airports, routine spraying with insecticide was carried out. For visitors arriving by train, they were inspected as they entered the colony. All immigrants entering by sea, air, or land were vaccinated against smallpox if they did not have valid vaccination certificates. In addition to these inspection and prophylactic vaccination duties, the administration was responsible for the maintenance of sanitary conditions in the port and airport, and the implementation of preventive measures against mosquitoes.[43]

Public medical services and personnel

It can be seen that during this period, Hong Kong had put in place an infra-structure and gradually expanded its capability to protect its residents from diseases, although many of the measures and programs were still limited in scope. Yet this concerted and extensive effort proved to be successful and would bear fruit by the second half of the 1960s when most of the infectious diseases were under control and an epidemiological transition took place. By the same token, the relative neglect of curative medical care during this period resulted in shortage of hospital beds and long lines at public hospitals waiting for medical consultation. Several factors accounted for the overloading of public clinic and hospital services, especially those related to out-patient care. There had been an increasing demand for Western medicine, even though Chinese medicine was still widely used; in fact, it was common for people to use both medical modalities when they were available. Second, government clinics and hospital out-patient services were low cost; and in the case of treating infectious diseases such as tuberculosis, medical care was usually free of charge. Third, health education and immunization campaigns had alerted the population to benefits of early detection of diseases and consequently more cases requiring medical attention were referred for treatment. The increase in demand and the pressure on medical services was revealed by the fact that in the period 1950–1962, first attendances at government out-patient centers rose by 154 percent, while the total population increased by approximately 65 percent.[44] The government relied heavily on the goodwill and cooperation of voluntary organizations and international philanthropic and religious agencies to offer low-cost medical care to those who could not afford private care.

Public medical care in postwar Hong Kong continued to be provided by government and government-assisted hospitals, clinics, and dispensaries. But only two new government hospitals were opened between 1945 and 1962. The Tsan Yuk Government Maternity Hospital was donated by the Royal Hong Kong Jockey Club and opened in 1954 and the other hospital was a mental hospital opened in 1961. In other words, despite the tremendous increase in demand, there were no additions of new general hospitals before 1962, except for the planned expansion of the largest general hospital, the Queen Mary Hospital, and the much delayed construction project of a new hospital in Kowloon that urgently needed more hospital facilities as the population continued to grow. Finally, in December 1963, the largest acute general hospital in Hong Kong, the Queen Elizabeth Hospital, became operational. General out-patient clinics were also planned and constructed, the first stages of which were completed in 1960–1961, with the opening of four clinics of varying size and scope of services. However, the government gave priority to the construction of specialized hospitals for infectious diseases, especially tuberculosis. Between 1949 and 1957, four hospitals for tuberculosis patients, including the Ruttonjee Sanatorium and the Grantham Hospital were opened. There were also tuberculosis out-patient clinics that provided care free of charge. Other institutions, for example, the Tung Wah Group Hospitals and the Alice Ho Miu Ling Nethersole Hospital, had roots before the war and continued to expand their work in the postwar years, serving especially the Chinese population and the poor.[45]

In view of the ever-increasing population and worsening environmental conditions, as well as the shortage of general hospital beds and out-patient facilities, a 15-year plan of development of medical and health services was drawn up in 1957. In planning for future developments, the underlying policy was "to provide additional hospital and clinic facilities for that part of the population that could not afford to pay economic charges for the services provided by private agencies." The government, of course, recognized that even this limited objective would involve a fairly sizable commitment of public funds since the assumption was that about 50 percent of the population would be dependent on government health services. The plan called for the doubling of hospital beds, from 2.67 per 1,000 of population in 1960 to 5.75 beds per 1,000 of population by 1965. It also recommended the construction of more clinics to provide both curative and preventive services. But before this proposal was finalized, the completion of several major projects, including the opening of the Queen Elizabeth Hospital, necessitated a reevaluation of the proposal, and the government decided to use the year 1963 as a new base line to develop a new proposal for the development of health services for the period 1963 to 1972.[46] The content of the new proposal and its implementation will be discussed in detail in the next chapter.

Not surprisingly, there was a shortage of qualified medical personnel in the immediate postwar period. The Japanese occupation forced many medical students to leave Hong Kong and make their way to Free China. Dr. Gordon King, Dean of Medicine at the University of Hong Kong also escaped to China and was instrumental in placing many of the students in Chinese medical schools that had set up operations in various cities in the interior of China. After the war, he also helped those students to secure the conferment of a Hong Kong degree. This group of wartime graduates who returned to Hong Kong proved to be invaluable in the rebuilding of Hong Kong's postwar medical infrastructure.[47]

The University of Hong Kong Medical School was the only medical school offering undergraduate medical training that was recognized by the General Medical Council of the UK. By 1960, between 35 and 50 students graduated each year – certainly too small a contingent to meet the urgent and huge demand from the growing population. Postgraduate education and training, however, was not available in the colony, and those medical graduates interested in additional professional training and research had to travel to the UK. As for the training of nurses, the addition of a new nursing school at the Queen Elizabeth Hospital, in addition to the one at Queen Mary Hospital, provided a much needed boost to the number of nursing personnel required to staff the hospitals and clinics being planned in the late 1950s and early 1960s. English was the medium of instruction in these two schools, while Chinese was used in the nurse training programs at the Tung Wah Hospitals, the Alice Ho Miu Ling Nethersole Hospital, and the Hong Kong Sanatorium and Hospital. The training of nurses in a hospital setting, instead of being part of an academic institution, would be the norm for some time to come. This modus operandi was in fact true of midwife training as well.[48]

The two decades after the war witnessed the remarkable recovery of Hong Kong and its transformation into a major manufacturing center while consolidating its position as a premier international trading port. As will be discussed in the next chapter, the policy of concentrating resources in combating infectious diseases had, by the second half of the 1960s, enabled Hong Kong to undergo an epidemiological transition characterized by the eradication or control of some of the major infectious diseases. At the same time, the government had become more interventionist in its social policy, whether in its attempts to deal with the refugee problem, or in the allocation of resources for social services. Toward the late 1960s, the changing demographics, the increasing demand for social amelioration from the poor, as well as the need to bolster the colonial regime's legitimacy would further necessitate a reorientation of the government's approach in its formulation and implementation of social services, including those targeting health care development and disease-control measures.

Notes

1 Frank Welsh, *A History of Hong Kong* (London: HarperCollins, 1997), 428–433.
2 Snow, *The Fall of Hong Kong: Britain, China and the Japanese Occupation*, 290.
3 Steve Tsang, "Government and politics in Hong Kong: a colonial paradox," in Judith M. Brown and Rosemary Foot eds., *Hong Kong's Transitions, 1842–1997* (London: MacMillan Press, 1997), 69–70; and Snow, *The Fall of Hong Kong*, 301.
4 Ting-Hong Wong, *Hegemonies Compared: State Formation and Chinese School Politics in Postwar Singapore and Hong Kong* (New York: Routledge, 2002), 108–110.
5 *The Economist*, November 4, 1999. From economist.com. Retrieved on August 12, 2015. See also Wm Roger Louis, "Hong Kong: the critical phrase, 1945–1949," *The American Historical Review*, 102:4 (October 1997), 1052–1084.
6 Alex H. Choi, "State-Business relations and industrial restructuring," in Ngo, *Hong Kong's History: State and Society under Colonial Rule*, 147–148.
7 Liu Shuyong, "Hong Kong: a survey of political and economic development over the past 150 years," *The China Quarterly*, 151 (September 1997), 583–589. See also Frank Leeming, "The earlier industrialization of Hong Kong," *Modern Asian Studies*, 9:3 (1975), 337–342.
8 T. D. Vaughan and D. J. Dwyer, "Some aspects of postwar population growth in Hong Kong," *Economic Geography*, 42:1 (January 1966), 38–39.
9 Quoted in Welsh, *A History of Hong Kong*, 445.
10 Ibid., 43. See also Sheila K. Johnson, "Hong Kong's resettled squatters: a statistical analysis," *Asian Survey*, 6:11 (November 1966), 643–656.
11 Johnson, "Hong Kong's resettled squatters," 644; and *Hong Kong Annual Report, 1952.*
12 For a discussion of the impact of the Shek Kip Mei fire on housing policy, see Alan Smart, *The Shek Kip Mei Myth: Squatters Fire and Colonial Rule in Hong Kong, 1950–1963* (Hong Kong: Hong Kong University Press, 2006). Margaret Jones has argued that in the prewar period, the Hong Kong government had already contemplated the idea of subsidizing housing out of government funds so as to improve living conditions of the Chinese population. This would, it was believed, control the spread of tuberculosis in the colony. See her "Tuberculosis, housing and the colonial state: Hong Kong, 1900–1950," 653–682.
13 Vaughan and Dwyer, "Some aspects of postwar population growth," 42. For interesting discussions of the squatter problem and resettlement policy, see D. J. Dwyer ed., *Asian Urbanization: A Hong Kong Casebook* (Hong Kong: Hong Kong University Press, 1971).
14 *Hong Kong Annual Reports 1950–51*, 26.
15 "Transfer of refugee soldiers," *Hong Kong Sunday Herald*, June 11, 1950; "Mount Davis refugees moved to new site at Junk Bay," *China Mail*, June 27, 1950.
16 Edvard Hambro, *The Problem of Chinese Refugees in Hong Kong: Report Submitted to the United Nations High Commission for Refugees* (Leyden: A. W. Sijthoff, 1955), 124.
17 Hu Yueh, "The Problem of the Hong Kong Refugees," *Asian Survey*, 2:1 (March 1962), 33–35; Hambro, *The Problem of Chinese Refugees in Hong Kong*; and Hong Kong Council of Social Services, *Meeting the Social Challenge: A Survey of the Work of Voluntary and Government Social Service Organization in Hong Kong* (Hong Kong: Hong Kong Council of Social Services, 1953).
18 *Hong Kong Annual Reports 1950–51*, 9; and *Hong Kong Annual Departmental Report by the Director of Medical and Health Services for the Financial Year 1960–61*, 1.
19 Ibid., 15, 18; and *Hong Kong Annual Departmental Report by the Director of Medical and Health Services for the Financial Year 1955–56*, 56–58.
20 *Development of Medical Services in Hong Kong* (Hong Kong: Government Printer, 1964), 3–4.

21 *Hong Kong Annual Departmental Report by the Director of Medical and Health Services for the Financial Year 1955–56*, 3.
22 *Hong Kong Annual Reports 1950–51*, Annexure G, 74.
23 Ibid.
24 A. S. Moodie, "Tuberculosis in Hong Kong," *Tubercle*, 44 (1962), 337.
25 *Hong Kong Annual Departmental Report by the Director of Medical and Health Services for the Financial Year 1955–56*, 15–16.
26 W. G. Allan, "Tuberculosis in Hong Kong, ten years later," *Tubercle*, 54:3 (1973), 236.
27 Ibid., 239–240; Moodie, "Tuberculosis in Hong Kong," 344; and *Hong Kong Annual Departmental Report by the Director of Medical and Health Services for the Financial Year 1955–56*, 14–15.
28 *Annual Report of the Hong Kong Anti-TB Association*, 1949 and 1960; *Hong Kong Annual Department Report by the Director of Medical and Health Services for the Financial Year 1960–61*.
29 Allan, "Tuberculosis in Hong Kong," 236.
30 S. H. Lee, "Malaria in Hong Kong," *Journal of Hong Kong Society of Community Medicine*, 15:1 (1985), 7.
31 *Hong Kong Annual Reports 1950–51*, 122.
32 Memo dated April 24, 1959, from the Director of Medical and Health Services to the Colonial Secretary, with enclosure. In Hong Kong Public Records Office, folder HKRS#41, D-S No. 1–9890.
33 *Hong Kong Annual Departmental Report by the Director of Medical and Health Services for the Financial Year 1960–61*, 35–38.
34 Ibid., 68; *Hong Kong Annual Reports 1950–51*, 23, 28; and *Hong Kong Annual Departmental Report by the Director of Medical and Health Services for the Financial Year 1955–56*, 67.
35 Frank Fenner, "Smallpox: emergence, global spread, and eradication," *History and Philosophy of the Life Sciences*, 15:3 (1993), 397–420.
36 *Hong Kong Annual Reports 1950–51*, 28; *Hong Kong Annual Departmental Report by the Director of Medical and Health Services for the Financial Year 1955–56*, 67; and *Hong Kong Annual Departmental Report by the Director of Medical and Health Services for the Financial Year 1960–61*, 18, 106.
37 *Hong Kong Annual Departmental Report by the Director of Medical and Health Services for the Financial Year 1955–56*, 6–7 and *Financial Year 1960–61*, 16–18. See also *The Urban Council, 1883–1983* (Hong Kong: The Urban Council, 1983); and Tsang, *A Documentary History of Hong Kong: Government and Politics*, 134–135.
38 Ibid., 8–10; and *Financial Year 1960–61*, 16–18. See also Lau, *A History of the Municipal Councils of Hong Kong, 1883–1999*.
39 *Hong Kong Annual Reports 1950–51*, 37–43. The quotes are from p. 43.
40 *Hong Kong Annual Departmental Report by the Director of Medical and Health Services for the Financial Year 1955–56*, 21–23; and *Financial Year 1960–61*, 43–45, 47.
41 *Hong Kong Annual Departmental Report by the Director of Medical and Health Services for the Financial Year 1955–56*, 23–24; *Financial Year 1960–61*, 45–46; and *Financial Year 1965–66*, 19.
42 *Hong Kong Annual Departmental Report by the Director of Medical and Health Services for the Financial Year 1960–61*, 46–47; and *Financial Year 1965–66*, 23–24.
43 *Hong Kong Annual Reports 1950–51*, 32; *Hong Kong Annual Departmental Report by the Director of Medical and Health Services for the Financial Year 1955–56*, 11–12; and *Financial Year 1960–61*, 41.
44 *Development of Medical Services in Hong Kong*, 4.
45 Ibid., 3–4; *Hong Kong Annual Reports 1950–51*, 80. *Hong Kong Annual Departmental Report by the Director of Medical and Health Services for the Financial Year 1960–61*, 48–58. See also Starling et al., *Plague, SRAS and the Story of Medicine*, 91–121.

46 *Development of Medical Services in Hong Kong*, 7–8. The quote is from p. 7.
47 Gordon King, "An episode in the history of the University," in Clifford Matthews and Oswald Cheung, *Dispersal and Renewal: Hong Kong University During the War Years* (Hong Kong: Hong Kong University Press, 1998).
48 *Hong Kong Annual Departmental Report by the Director of Medical and Health Services for the Financial Year 1960–61*, 77–79.

6 Epidemiological transition and disease prevention, 1960s–1980s

The citation conferring the Honorary Doctor of Law degree on Sir David Trench at the 69th Congregation (1968) of the University of Hong Kong noted that Sir David had led Hong Kong "out of the woods last summer," and that "instead of resting on his laurels," he had been "looking forward, planning for our future."[1] Trench's governorship, from April 1964 to October 1971 was challenged not only by social disturbances – the most serious being the riots in the summer of 1967 referred to in the citation – but also by changing political realities as well as social and economic developments that made it necessary for the colonial government to re-evaluate its policies in order to maintain social and political stability as well as sustained economic growth. Trench was able to weather the crisis in 1967 and, with an eye to improving relations with the public, introduced measures designed to give the government a more active role in social reforms. These included the city district office scheme, civil service reforms, labor legislations, and an effort to make Chinese an official language.[2] Murray MacLehose, Trench's successor, also initiated or broadened reforms that would have a direct impact on the colony's socio-economic developments, including its health care policies. By the early 1970s, the most violent phase of China's Cultural Revolution was history and with China's rapprochement with the US, cross-border relations stabilized. Moreover, Deng Xiaoping's plans to modernize China and the opening of Special Economic Zones, the first being Shenzhen in 1980 just across the border of Hong Kong reinforced the significance of the "China Factor" in almost all aspects of Hong Kong's development, not the least of which was its health policies and disease prevention as increased cross-border travel would inevitably facilitate the spread of contagions in the entire region. At the same time, toward the end of MacLehose's tenure, the questions surrounding Hong Kong's political future – and its economic and social prospects – emerged as the most critical factor shaping the triangular relationship of Britain, China, and Hong Kong. MacLehose would in fact play a crucial role in preparing the stage for Sino-British negotiations over Hong Kong's future after he left office in May 1982.

Moving forward: 1960s to 1980s

As before, the formulation and implementation of health policies were to a significant extent affected by political and socio-economic developments during this period, one which was marked by rapid economic expansion, widening income inequalities, population growth, and the emergence of a young postwar generation less prone to accept the status quo. Postwar reconstruction in the 1950s and early 1960s had not only brought about Hong Kong's recovery but also the colony's economic restructuring: from entrepot trade to manufacturing, service, and finance during the 1960s to 1980s. At the same time, economic prosperity brought into focus once again some of the major issues that the colony had been grappling with since the early postwar period: taking care of the growing population, especially the poorer segment of the population that constituted the bulk of the manufacturing labor force, and providing appropriate social services short of turning Hong Kong into a welfare state; and the need as well as the means to maintain a healthy labor force that would help to sustain economic growth in a period of industrialization and restructuring.

As we have seen, despite wartime destruction, Hong Kong successfully transformed itself into a manufacturing center in the 1950s and early 1960s, thanks to the business acumen of entrepreneurs from China and a pool of cheap labor provided by the huge influx of refugees. Yet in the 1970s and early 1980s, Hong Kong's export-led economic strategy was increasingly challenged by Taiwan and South Korea. Moreover, with China's launching of the Four Modernizations and "opening," factories began to relocate across the border to take advantage of lower labor and land costs. The percentage of the labor force in manufacturing declined from about 40 in 1980 to 30 in 1989.[3] However, the business community adjusted to the new situation by moving into financial and business services, taking advantage of Hong Kong's excellent banking facilities and growing foreign direct investment: Hong Kong was emerging as an international financial center.

Not everyone, however, shared in Hong Hong's economic prosperity, especially in the first two decades after the war. In fact, despite some increases in household incomes, income inequalities in the colony sharpened and studies have shown that "in 1966, income inequality in Hong Kong was its worst ever."[4] Beginning in April 1966, protests over a fare increase of the cross-harbor Star ferry led to demonstrations and riots in Kowloon, resulting in the death of one person shot by the police. The fare increase served as the incident that galvanized a younger postwar generation willing to openly challenge the relative deprivation that they and others suffered amidst growing prosperity: the deplorable housing and working conditions and a government seemingly insensitive to their plight. In fact, the *Report of Commission of Inquiry* pointed out that this younger generation, unlike their elders, were ready to demand change and it cautioned the government to provide opportunities and ways for the younger people to participate in community life and to open up channels of communication with the community.[5] More unrest erupted in May the following year, this time politically inspired by the Cultural Revolution in China. An industrial dispute in a factory in Kowloon led to the intervention of the communist-dominated Federation of Trade Unions, and local communist elements mobilized in an anti-colonial movement that was marked by demonstrations, strikes, riots, and bomb explosions. Many newspapers and local organizations, including the *kaifongs* supported the government's firm but measured actions to deal with the situation, including the banning of communist newspapers and the de-registration of a communist-controlled school. By late 1967, relative calm had returned to Hong Kong.[6]

The social turmoil of 1966 and 1967 proved to be critical in alerting the government to the urgent need to reappraise its socio-economic policy, and take the initiative to enhance the legitimacy of colonial rule. The pressing issues confronting the government that had the greatest impact on the population remained to be housing and social service reforms.

Housing and new towns

Housing, proclaimed the *1971 Hong Kong Annual Review*, the first to be issued under MacLehose's influence, was "a key to so much – health, family solidarity, community spirit, distribution of labour, communications needs, to name a few factors only."[7] Indeed, we have seen that it was a concern that significantly impacted the government's formulation of social service and health policies since the end of the war. In the 1950s, the rising population as well as the issue of squatters and overcrowded tenements had already contributed to the government's decision to construct resettlement estates and public housing. But the problems of housing, sanitation, and social service improvements in general persisted. The pressure of population growth never let up, thanks to the continual influx of immigrants from the mainland. The first postwar census in 1961 recorded a population of about 3.1 million, compared to about 2.2 million in the mid-1950s. Significantly, 40.8 percent of the population was under 15 years old, while 16 percent was under five years old. This age structure pointed to a potential dramatic population growth from 1965 onwards owing to a potential jump in the rate of natural increase as the 15-year-old and younger elements started to become parents.[8] At the same time, the rate of immigration remained high until late 1980 when the colonial government discontinued the "touch base" immigration policy. By the mid-1980s, Hong Kong's population had reached an estimated 5.4 million. Not surprisingly, population pressure and changing demographics not only called into question the viability of some of the social service and health care policies initiated in the 1950s, but also created new issues and concerns that forced the government to adjust policy orientations especially in housing and health.

In the 1950s and early 1960s, the squatter population included not only immigrants and refugees from the mainland but also many of the city's poor, struggling to survive. As noted, in the second half of the 1950s, the government's housing policy focused on the construction of resettlement estates laid out in typical back-to-back "H blocks." Family units were tiny and residents had to share sanitary facilities.[9] Compounding the problems was the shortage of water, a situation that had a devastating impact on the housing situation and sanitation in the colony as a whole. In the older estates, many families had to share one kitchen with a single tap, which, because of restrictions, might supply water for only several hours per day. Since 1963, the water situation had become critical, and private residents received water once every four days and only for one period of four hours. From 1964 to 1967, two new reservoirs were constructed: the Shek Pik Scheme (on Lantau Island) in 1964, and the Plover Cove in Tolo Harbor in 1967. But they were not able to meet the needs of the growing population and Hong Kong had to purchase water of the East River across the border.[10]

Critics however, charged that even the new estates were no better than the substandard back-to-back prewar tenement houses. In 1963, the government appointed a Working Party to investigate the conditions of the squatters and re-evaluate resettlement policies. The *Report of the 1963 Working Party on Government Policies and Practices with regard to Squatters, Resettlement and Government Low Cost Housing* made it clear that the government's "rosy" picture of new accommodation for the rising population was not tenable; in fact, the report pointed to a grave problem that had been overlooked: viz., conditions in many of the postwar tenements were so deplorable that their residents should be considered for relocation just as the squatters. It concluded that the ever-increasing numbers of tenants and sub-tenants in postwar buildings "may well present a more serious health hazard, and bring up their children mentally, socially and physically more handicapped or stunted" than if they were in the squatter areas.[11]

As early as the 1950s, with the setting up of an industrial satellite town at Kwun Tong, the government had entertained the idea of population dispersal by developing new towns in peripheral locations outside of existing built-up areas. The establishment of the first generation of new towns, however, took place in the 1960s and early 1970s: Tsun Wan was designated as a new town in 1960, Shatin in 1967, and Tuen Mun in 1967. When MacLehose became governor, he further committed the government to a 10-year housing program aimed at providing housing for 1.8 million people. The proactive approach resulted in the establishment of four more high-density, high-rise new towns between 1979 and 1982. The decentralization of these new population centers in the New Territories was designed to not only ease urban overcrowding, but also improve the social, environmental, and health care pressure experienced by the already congested existing urban centers – pressure that had contributed to social instability as witnessed in the disturbances in the mid-1960s. By 1981, almost 1 million people called these new towns home.[12]

These towns were originally conceived as self-contained living and working spaces with balanced land-use, and they generally included industrial development as part of the planning. To attract residents, public housing of various types was built, and they were improvements over the older H block estates, including amenities such as private sanitary facilities and recreational areas. There was also housing for middle-income families constructed by private developers.[13] The establishment of these new towns resulted in the gradual and continual urbanization of the once rural and mostly thinly populated New Territories. Not surprisingly, the government had to pay increasing attention to the issues of sanitation, disease control, and health of the bourgeoning population in these new urban centers.

Industrialization, urban services, and health protection

The rapid industrialization in the 1960s and early 1970s created new health problems for the colony. One of the objectives of the establishment of new towns was to provide industrial and residential centers that would generate ample manufacturing and employment opportunities for their residents. The initial results, however, proved to be disappointing as the lack of infra-structure and adequate transportation deterred many industries from relocating; and with insufficient opportunities, many residents found it easier to commute to nearby urban centers for employment.[14] For most of the factories in old built-up areas – many of them small family concerns – they had to deal with aggravated problems of congestion, environmental hygiene, occupational hazards, and industrial accidents among the work force.[15] Working conditions in these factories were harsh and workers often lived in poverty.

There was another pressing issue: to augment their incomes, many workers found it necessary to not only work in factories but also turn their tiny apartments into workshops of all kinds, a development that had also emerged in prewar Hong Kong's early industrialization. Securing subcontract orders for piece work provided additional income for family members, including children who participated in the manufacturing of toys, plastic flowers, and garments. Unfortunately, hygienic conditions in these tiny shops were in most cases deplorable, especially when many of them lacked adequate sanitary facilities and safety provisions. But household production contributed sig-nificantly to Hong Kong's economic prosperity and regulatory laxity on the part of the government enabled these flexible and exploitative labor practices to continue in the 1960s and 1970s. Not surprisingly, civil disturbances in the mid-1960s erupted against a background of widening social inequalities and increasing dissatisfaction among the underclass with the appalling living and working conditions.

Both Governors Trench and MacLehose were keenly aware of the importance of improving working and living conditions for the working class to ensure a healthy labor force, social stability, and economic growth. Government expenditures on social services for labor increased from HK$4 million in 1967–1968 to HK$18.7 million in 1976–1977.[16] In 1964, occupational diseases were brought under the Workmen's Compensation Ordinance for the first time. Compensations for incapacity and death were raised the following year.[17]

Under Trench and MacLehose, the Ordinance was amended several times to increase the amount of compensation and add new benefits, including medical and surgical allowances for injured workers.[18] The Industrial Health Service was responsible for the evaluation of occupational injuries and disabilities of workers.[19]

With increased urbanization and the rapid expansion of industrial and residential developments, the adequate provision of such urban services as environmental sanitation, waste collection, water supply and cleanliness, maintenance of public latrines and public places, and health inspection became essential to disease prevention and health protection. In the early 1960s, the Urban Council's Hygiene Division had a number of health inspectors responsible for sanitary inspection of domestic dwellings as well as premises licensed by the Council, supervision of markets, investigation into cases of notified disease and disinfection of premises, and popular health education. The Cleansing division took care of refuse collection and disposal, and street cleaning and washing.[20] The Council summed up its main duties very well in its 1968/69 report: "The main purpose of the department is to ensure the maintenance of adequate standards of public health."[21] In 1973, the Urban Council was reorganized and gained financial autonomy; while it continued to be concerned with urban services related to public health, all matters related to housing were now under the jurisdiction of the Housing Authority.

Epidemiological transition and communicable diseases

Construction of resettlement estates – though not entirely satisfactory – and population dispersal, as well as expanded urban services had helped to alleviate somewhat the health problems associated with the squatters and overcrowded old tenements. At the same time, the government had, as we have seen, concentrated the lion's share of health resources during the first two decades after the war on developing public health programs to combat epidemics and communicable diseases. The objective of course was to create a healthy environment for economic growth and to prevent outbreaks of disease subject to international quarantine in order to ensure Hong Kong's economic survival.

The government's policy paid off; by the second half of the 1960s, a modern epidemiological profile emerged. The concept of epidemiological transition posits "the transition from a cause of death pattern dominated by infectious diseases with very high mortality, especially at younger ages, to a pattern dominated by chronic diseases and injuries with lower mortality, mostly peaking at older ages, that is seen to be responsible for the tremendous increase in life expectancy."[22] Based on this framework, Hong Kong has "provided one of the most spectacular and complete examples of epidemiological transition."[23] The transition is evident from vital statistics of the crude death rate (per 1,000 population), infant mortality (per 1,000 live births), and maternal mortality (per 1,000 total births) from 1960 to 1985. The crude death rate declined from 6.4 in 1960, to 5.3 in 1970, and to 4.7 in 1985. The infant mortality rate also dropped from 41.5 in 1960, to 19.6 in 1970, to 7.6 in 1985. Finally, maternal mortality also declined from 0.49 in 1960 to 0.19 in 1970 to 0.05 in 1985.[24] Thanks to the general improvement in environmental hygiene and the success in the provision of governmental maternal and child health services, there had been a rapid decline of the infant mortality rate; and by 1975, the rate of 15.0 per thousand live births was "at a lower level than many European and American countries."[25] Moreover, Hong Kong's crude death rate of 4.9 percent in 1975 compared very favorably with those of Japan (6.4 percent), United Kingdom (11.9 percent), and US (8.9 percent) in the same year.

There was also a transition in the main causes of death: viz., decreasing mortality from infectious and febrile diseases and increases in deaths from such diseases as neoplasms, heart disease and diseases associated with aging. There had been a steady decline in infectious and parasitic diseases during the period from 1960 to 1975: from 14.4 percent of total deaths in 1960, to 10.0 percent in 1965, 7.0 percent in 1970, and 4.0 percent in 1975. On the other hand, there had been a relative and in some cases absolute increase in degenerative diseases. Neoplasms, for example, accounted for 10.5 percent of total deaths in 1960, 18.1 in 1965, 19.1 percent in 1970, and 24.2 percent in 1975, a fairly typical trend for a developed country. In fact, deaths caused by carcinoma of the lung exceeded those from tuberculosis for the first time in 1973. Age-specific mortality rates also revealed the changes, especially among the elderly, with their major causes of death being neoplasms and heart disease.[26] Dr. G.H. Choa, Director of Medical and Health Services summed up the changing situation succinctly in his 1970–1971 annual departmental report: "the Colony is facing increasing problems arising from non-communicable diseases. The major causes of death are cancer, heart and hypertensive diseases, pneumonia, cerebrovascular lesions and tuberculosis. The effects of industrialization and urbanization together with the ageing of a relatively young population have added problems for the care of the sick and disabled."[27]

Of course, the decline in incidences of communicable and infectious diseases did not mean that they had been wiped out. As we have seen, smallpox, however, was an exception, thanks to the vigorous mass vaccination campaign against the disease. In July 1979, Hong Kong was certified to be smallpox free by the WHO. Despite the fact that the government's policy of prioritizing the control of infectious diseases in the two decades after the war was generally successful, problems caused by several infectious and communicable diseases persisted. There were also newly emerging diseases such as HIV/AIDS in the 1980s. Malaria had been one of the major infectious diseases that were targeted by the government in its concerted public health program. Anti-larval operations, as well as sanitary improvements in general proved to be crucial in reducing the incidence of malaria; at the same time, the rapid urbanization of Hong Kong and most of Kowloon vastly reduced the natural habitat of mosquitoes. But the New Territories remained quite malarious as people moving to the new towns and outlying areas were venturing into areas where malaria transmission was still quite prevalent and vector control programs were only beginning in the early 1960s.[28] Health education, epidemiological surveillance, and constant monitoring of cases also contributed to the success of the overall anti-malaria efforts. The Malaria Bureau continued its research in malaria transmission and conducted mosquito surveys and malaria surveys. Local malaria transmission was finally interrupted in 1969 and no local case due to natural transmission was reported in 1970.[29] In fact, except for imported cases, for example among Vietnamese refugees who arrived in Hong Kong in the second half of the 1970s, Hong Kong became virtually free from malaria from the 1970s onward.[30]

Hong Kong also became relatively free from another major infectious disease, cholera, by the second half of the 1960s, but not before two serious outbreaks in 1961 and 1964. The chronic exiguous water supply and unsanitary conditions in parts of Hong Kong provided favorable conditions for potential contamination of food and water. Moreover, the sizable boat population living on junks and sampans were particularly vulnerable to often-polluted marine environment and unsanitary conditions. In mid-August 1961, cases of a new subtype of cholera called cholera El Tor were reported, marking the beginning of an epidemic lasting until the end of September. A total of 129 cases were recorded with more than 700 contacts isolated in a quarantine center. The highest incidence rate, 30 percent of the cases, was among the boat people. The government acted quickly to provide territory-wide free inoculation at a number of stations and mobile inoculation teams were dispatched to outlying areas. Public response was overwhelming and the government had to request fresh supplies of vaccines from elsewhere. Health inspectors intensified their efforts in enforcing sanitary and cleanliness regulations in markets, food stalls, and water supplies. The last confirmed case appeared on September 23, and on October 12, Hong Kong was declared free from cholera infection.[31]

The cholera outbreak in Hong Kong was part of the seventh cholera pandemic that spread from Indonesia in 1961 and reached Hong Kong in August. The pandemic actually continued to extend to western Pakistan, Afghanistan, Iran, southern USSR, and Iraq from 1964–1966. Countries affected by the outbreak faced international quarantine and Hong Kong was no exception. After Hong Kong was declared an infected port, a number of neighboring countries immediately placed restrictions on the export of certain foodstuffs from Hong Kong. The outbreak again revealed the vulnerability of Hong Kong as the constant movement of people, especially from the mainland, would easily help to spread pathogens if they originated across the border. In fact, the infection was suspected to have come to Hong Kong from Guangdong Province. One of the recommendations of the official report on the outbreak was the creation of a regional liaison with the neighboring territories affected by the outbreak, including Guangdong and Macau. Moreover, to prevent future outbreaks, the government was urged to have time-specific inoculation campaigns beginning in February, March, and April the following year while health education efforts were to be redoubled.[32]

The other cholera outbreak occurred in May 1964. Although it was of short duration, yet it proved once again the importance of vigilance in maintaining a clean water supply and high standards of food hygiene in face of the ease with which a water-borne cholera epidemic could break out. The outbreak was traced to a restaurant owner's unlawful connection of the well-water storage tank with the mains water storage tank that provided potable water to the kitchen in the restaurant, resulting in the contamination of the water supply. There were 14 cases of cholera and four of the patients died.[33] Although there were no major outbreaks in the 1970s and 1980s, cholera continued to be a health threat because of visits of infected international travelers and local residents who had visited infected places and developed symptoms after returning to Hong Kong.

The cholera pandemic of 1961 was not the only pandemic of communicable diseases that affected Hong Kong during this period. The Hong Kong flu pandemic of 1968 was the third influenza pandemic to occur in the twentieth century and originated in China. In Hong Kong, the epidemic broke out in mid-July 1968, reaching its maximum intensity in late July and lasted for about six weeks. The high population density in urban areas certainly facilitated the spread of the highly contagious virus; altogether about 500,000 persons, or 15 percent of the population were affected. Fortunately, symptoms were mild and there were no excess deaths during the epidemic. But within several months of the outbreak in Hong Kong, the virus spread swiftly throughout Southeast Asia, then the US and the United Kingdom, much of Europe, and in 1969, reached Japan, South Africa, and South America.[34] The cholera pandemic and influenza pandemic in the 1960s revealed the potential of widespread epidemic and indeed pandemic outbreaks as Hong Kong emerged as a global city and the process of globalization accelerated in the next few decades.

Despite steady success in the control of tuberculosis in the two decades after the war, the disease still remained one of the leading causes of death during this period although infant mortality from the disease had declined to virtually nil in 1971, thanks to the government's policy of BCG vaccination of newborns. But in 1965, "the estimated incidence of 1.5 percent of adults with active disease [was]...amongst the highest in the world."[35] Since it was virtually impossible, physically and financially, to provide institutional accommodation for the sick, the government focused on the out-patient treatment of patients through chest clinics, including several in the rural areas, whose staff also conducted home visits and contact tracing. By the 1970s, hospital admissions were reserved only for serious cases, and the program was freely available to all without qualification. With general improvements in housing and working conditions as well as a rise in the living standard, the tuberculosis death rate gradually declined by the 1970s, although the notification rate remained fairly high as a result of increased public awareness of the disease, constant improvements in case finding and the continual influx of refugees and immigrants from neighboring areas. The tuberculosis death rate fell from 14.8 percent per

100,000 population in 1975 to 9.1 percent in 1978; by 1985, it fell to 7.5 percent.[36] It should be pointed out that the general improvement in living standards and conditions in the 1970s had helped to reduce the infection rate. As tuberculosis mortality gradually declined, the main institutions initially designated to accommodate tuberculosis patients, notably the Ruttonjee Sanatorium and Grantham Hospital, were converted respectively into a general district hospital and cardio-thoracic center.

What is worrisome, however, is that as early as the mid-1960s, there was already a high incidence of tuberculosis drug resistance.[37] This had the potential of chronic positive patients spreading the infection. Doctors in Hong Kong began using a combination of various drugs for several months since 1979 and the method had since been generally adopted worldwide.[38] But multidrug resistant tuberculosis (MDR-TB) emerged as a most serious problem by the 2000s, especially in countries such as China, Brazil, India, the Russian Federation, and South Africa. The general breakdown of the health care system in China since the 1980s contributed to not only a large tuberculosis epidemic but also a high incidence of MDR-TB.[39] Hong Kong had to be constantly on the alert for the potential spread of MDR-TB from China and other countries.

Public health services

Much of the success in reducing or eliminating the threat of major diseases and epidemics resulted from the concerted efforts to control communicable diseases in the first two decades after the war as well as in the continuation and expansion of public health services and the consolidations and establishment of new ones even after the government's health policy shifted to prioritizing curative medical services since the mid-1960s. The steady decline in infant mortality, for example, owed much to the continual growth of the programs of the Maternal and Child Health Services (later renamed Family Health Services) which, by early 1980s, not only provided ante-natal and post-natal care for mothers, but also family planning counseling. Moreover, immunization programs were conducted against tuberculosis, diphtheria, whooping cough, tetanus, poliomyelitis, measles, and rubella.[40]

The government continued to place great emphasis on the pre-teen and teen population. The work of the earlier school health service continued; these included preventive work, sanitary inspection of school premises, and health education propaganda. A School Medical Service was inaugurated in September 1964 to provide medical examinations of children in specific ages and referring those requiring attention to clinics and immunization programs. Although school participation was voluntary, demand for the services steadily increased; in 1983, 300,000 school children – representing about 39 percent of the total eligible school population – from 783 schools participated in the scheme.[41]

The role of the Port Health Service in protecting Hong Kong from the introduction of quarantinable diseases became even more critical in the 1970s and 1980s as Hong Kong became an international financial center, as well as one of the busiest ports and tourist sites in Asia. While it protected Hong Kong from imported diseases, it also prevented communicable diseases from being carried away from Hong Kong. The arrival of thousands of Vietnamese refugees (boat people) beginning in the second half of the 1970s, many of whom were from areas where plague and cholera were endemic, would seriously challenge the capability of the service to keep Hong Kong free from communicable diseases.[42]

Medical services and adjustment of health policy

The control of most communicable diseases by the second half of the 1960s and early 1970s was achieved, however, at the expense of curative medical services. Not enough attention, and resources, had been given to the construction of medical facilities, including hospitals and clinics, despite the fact that an increasing number of people were seeking Western biomedical treatments for their ailments. The government's policy had been dictated by several considerations: first, it would not, and could not, provide comprehensive medical care to the entire population; second, it would, however, make available hospital and clinic facilities to the needy who did not have the means to seek medical help from private providers; third, as in the case of the provision of public health services, housing, or education, improvements and initiatives had to be economically sustainable.[43] Fortunately, those reforms were supported by an economic expansion that, in fact, took place in the 1970s and 1980s. With the fiscal constraints imposed by the government, private and community organizations such as the *kaifongs* as well as international philanthropic and religious agencies were encouraged to play an increasingly greater role in offering low cost care. In 1966, 96 percent of the 29 *kaifongs* in Hong Kong ran some form of medical clinics.[44] Certainly, some sought relief from practitioners of traditional Chinese medicine who, however, were not recognized by the government and remained outside the official medical service system until after 1997.[45] At the same time, the colonial government had often accentuated one of the key elements in Chinese culture – the importance of family obligations and self-reliance – to encourage the family to assume more responsibility for the medical care of its members.[46]

For those seeking help from government clinics or hospitals, long queues and lengthy waits were the rule. There was also a serious shortage of hospital beds for the growing population; as noted in the last chapter, between 1954 and 1961, only two new hospitals – the Tsan Yuk Maternity hospital and the Castle Peak Mental hospital – were built.[47] An earlier plan developed in 1957 to develop medical and health services was replaced by a new plan that used 1963 as the base line for proposed new initiatives. The Medical Development Plan for the period 1963–1973 to address the inadequacy of facilities, and to plan for future needs was a major attempt to anticipate future needs in health care. The White Paper, entitled *Developments of Medical Services in Hong*

Kong, issued in 1964, stressed the importance of health to Hong Kong's economic growth: "a good general standard of health throughout a community is an economic asset to it and helps to condition the levels of energy and initiative which determines productivity, particularly in a free enterprise economy, such as Hong Kong."[48] The government's policy was to ensure that the estimated 50 percent of the community that could not pay for out-patient treatment would receive care – free or through subsidy – in government hospitals and clinics.[49] Yet the provision of care was, as before, subject to the availability of resources.

The White Paper projected that more hospital beds were urgently needed. In December 1963, the ratio of all types of beds, including those for infectious diseases, per 1,000 population was 3.13, and the study recommended a ratio of 4.25 by 1972.[50] It also pointed to the changing population distribution as a factor to be considered in determining future locations of new hospitals. The opening of Queen Elizabeth Hospital, the largest acute general hospital in the city in December 1963 certainly helped to ease the pressure on hospital care in Kowloon and the New Territories. As for the provision of out-patient services in government clinics, the study again stressed the need to open more centers in Kowloon to take care of the growing population. Indeed, with the development of new towns, there was a marked deficiency in easily accessible clinics.[51]

As we have seen, the government, responding to the social unrest in the second half of the 1960s, had become more proactive in social service reforms. Steady progress was made to remedy the problems of public medical services as recommended by the 1963 White Paper. A number of projects involving the construction of new hospital wings and wards as well as general and specialty clinics were begun or completed by 1971.[52] As far as the increase in hospital beds was concerned, the government was able to meet the recommendation of the 1963 study, as the ratio was 4.26 at the end of 1972.[53] Although patients could choose between public, subvented, or private hospitals, and government or private clinics, most relied on government facilities as the fees were much lower, even though the problems of long queues, lengthy waiting times, and the use of temporary beds in hospitals had actually worsened as the demand for Western medicine continued to increase among the growing population.

Since the 1963 White Paper dealt with proposed developments of public medical services up to 1973, the government issued another study, entitled *The Further Development of Medical and Health Services in Hong Kong* in July 1974 to review past developments and to recommend improvements and appropriate expansion for the next decade. In addition to addressing the deficiencies in the existing system, some of the new realities that the study took into consideration included the continual urbanization of the New Territories, the expansion of new towns, the expected population growth, the epidemiological transition, and the health problems of the elderly. The study recommended the adoption of a regional approach to coordinate and administer medical and health services; each region would have a regional hospital with specialized care, one or more district hospitals for non-specialized care, a number of general clinics, and one or more specialist clinics or polyclinics. Patients would be channeled to the appropriate level of care without clotting the out-patient departments or Accidents and Emergency Departments of hospitals. The study claimed that the integrated network of services in a common geographical area would ensure a more even utilization of medical and health resources, better facilities in the urban areas, and more effective coverage of clinic services throughout Hong Kong. Four regions would be set up initially, and a fifth was to be added later to serve East New Territories.[54]

The implementation of this plan, however, was not as smooth as envisioned. Voluntary hospitals could refuse to join the scheme and to accept uniform bed-pricing policy. Not surprisingly, since government hospitals normally charged lower fees than other hospitals, most patients were reluctant to be moved to a more expensive institution. Conflicts over resources existed between hospitals within a region, and there were also management problems related to the new civil service staff placed in regional offices that possessed little experience of hospital administration and tended to be inflexible in the resolution of problems.[55] By the end of 1983, the projected 10-year period covered by the study, the ratio of hospital beds: 4.3 to 1,000 population, was about the same as that of 1972. The Director of Medical and Health Services indeed reported that "pressure on the service was experienced on all fronts, reflected by the increase in attendance at out-patient clinics, accident and emergency departments and by the number of hospital admissions."[56] More reforms might be needed.

Medical and health personnel

One of the recommendations of the 1974 White Paper was the establishment of a second medical school at the Chinese University of Hong Kong. The shortage of physicians of Western medicine had become critical from the 1970s onward as the demand for Western medicine surged. With inadequate governmental facilities providing care, charitable or religious organizations, *kaifongs*, and the Tung Wah Group of Hospitals offered much-needed relief through their clinics or hospitals. Maryknoll, for example, managed clinics in Kwun Tong.[57] And, as noted, *kaifongs* also provided some sort of general medical services for residents in their respective communities.[58]

The recommendation for the establishment of a second physician-training institution was therefore timely as the intake of students to the colony's only medical school at the University of Hong Kong remained low: 79 in 1963–1964; and by the 1970s, the number increased to 150 per year.[59] The government finally approved the establishment of a new medical school in 1974, and the first class of students was admitted in 1981. In a speech given in 1978, Choh-Ming Li, the founding Vice-Chancellor of the Chinese University of Hong Kong remarked that the new medical students would be reminded of the 1974 White Paper's recommendation for an additional 100 doctors per year for the medical and health services, and hence their "future roles in the public services."[60]

To meet the immediate needs for additional physicians, the government decided, amidst much opposition, to recruit a large number of unregistered doctors to staff the Medical and Health Department in late 1974. A compromise was finally reached between the government and the Hong Kong Medical Association representing the registered doctors: non-Commonwealth doctors would have to pass an examination and complete an 18-month "externship" (clinical attachment) to be registered. This would allow the government to have a pool of registered doctors within a relatively short period of time. The solution, however, did not solve the fundamental flaw in the colony's utilization and distribution of medical personnel. Government and government-assisted hospitals provided almost 90 percent of the total hospital beds in the city, yet they hired only about 30 percent of the total number of doctors. Not surprisingly, the more attractive remuneration packages and working conditions offered by private institutions succeeded in creating an imbalance in the availability of physician care.[61]

The training of other medical and health personnel gradually expanded during this period. Since Hong Kong did not have a Dental School until 1980 when it was established in the University of Hong Kong, the government had been sending students with scholarships to receive training overseas. Dental technicians were trained locally, while dental surgery assistants and dental nurses were also sent overseas for training.[62] As for nurse training, the number of government hospital schools of nursing increased to three in 1970, and by early 1984, there were eight such schools for general registered nurses with an annual enrollment of about 1,200 nurses a year. Post-graduate training was available locally or overseas, while two-year courses for nursing auxiliaries helped to augment nursing staff in routine basic nursing care.[63] The expanded number of health personnel was sorely needed as the public health and medical services expanded both numerically and spatially during this period. The situation, by the beginning of the 1980s, was summed up by Dr. K.L. Thong, the Director of Medical and Health Services: "the ever-increasing population, the rising expectation of the people coupled with the constraints of limited financial and manpower resources have imposed a heavy strain on the provision of these services. Attendances at all the existing health care centres had been on the increase and attained record heights."[64] The search for a viable health policy would continue; indeed, since the recommendations of the 1974 White Paper only covered the decade to 1984, new initiatives would be needed to meet the challenges of the next decade.

The 1960s–1980s was a critical period in Hong Kong history. The government's almost single-minded dedication to fostering economic growth in the 1960s had contributed to the growing economic prosperity, although it was not shared by the poorer segments of the population. The turning point came after the social disturbances in the mid-1960s when the government adopted a more proactive stance in increasing investments in social and welfare programs in education, housing, and medical services. This policy was continued through the 1970s under the governorship of MacLehose who in fact, was able to project a positive and benevolent image to solidify public support for the administration. In the midst of unprecedented economic growth and social stability, MacLehose was certainly well aware of the uncertainty surrounding the impending retrocession, due in 1997, and its impact on Hong Kong's future. His trip to China in 1979 proved pivotal to the negotiations between Beijing and London over the future of the city. As far as social and health care policies in the 1980s and 1990s were concerned, much would indeed depend on the outcome of the negotiations leading to retrocession.

Notes

1 "The University of Hong Kong: The Honorary Graduates, 69th Congregation (1968): Sir David Clive Crosbie Trench, Doctor of Laws *honoris causa*" from http://www4.hku.hk/hongrads/index.php/archive/graduate_detail/137. Retrieved on March 11, 2015.
2 Hsin-chi Kuan, "Political Stability and Change in Hong Kong," *International Journal of Sociology,* 9:3 (Fall 1979), 121–142; Timothy Man Kong Wong, "The Changing Meanings of Governorship in Hong Kong between 1946 and 1997; with Reference to the China Factor in Hong Kong," *Hong Kong Journal of Modern Chinese History,* 1 (2003), 121–122.
3 Liu, "Hong Kong: A survey of political and economic development," 589; and Yasheng Huang, "The Economic and Political Integration of Hong Kong: Implications for Government-Business Relations," in Warren Cohen and Li Zhao eds., *Hong Kong Under Chinese Rule. The Economic and Political Implications of Reversion* (Cambridge: Cambridge University Press, 1997), 102.
4 Zhao Xiaobin, Zhang Li, and Sit Tak O. Kelvin, "Income inequalities under economic restructuring in Hong Kong," *Asian Survey,* 44:3 (May/June 2004), 442–473. The quote is from p. 452. See also Irene Eng, "Flexible production in late industrialization: the case of Hong Kong," *Economic Geography,* 73:1 (January 1997), 26–43.
5 Hong Kong Government, Commission of Inquiry, *Kowloon Disturbances 1966: Report of Commission of Inquiry* (Hong Kong: Government Printer, 1967).
6 For the official account of the 1967 disturbances, see *Hong Kong Disturbances, 1967* (Hong Kong Government Printer, 1968); see also Ray Yep, "The 1967 riots in Hong Kong: the diplomatic and domestic fronts of the colonial governor," *The China Quarterly,* 193 (March 2008), 122–139; Gary Ka-Wai Cheung, *Hong Kong's Watershed: The 1967 Riots* (Hong Kong: Hong Kong University Press, 2009); and Zhang Jiawei (Cheung Ka-wai), *Xianggang 67 baodong neijing* [The inside story of the 1967 riot in Hong Kong] (Hong Kong: Pacific Century Press Ltd., 2000).
7 Quoted in Welsh, *A History of Hong Kong,* 478.
8 Vaughan and Dwyer, "Some Aspects of Population Growth in Hong Kong," 41.
9 Ibid., 43.
10 *Hong Kong Fact Sheets – Water, Power, Gas Supplies* from www.gov.hk/en/about/a bouthk/factsheets/docs/wp&g-supplies.pdf. Retrieved on March 30, 2015.
11 Working Party on Government Policies and Practices, *Report of the 1963 Working Party on Government Policies and Practices with regards to Squatters, Resettlement and Government Low Cost Housing* (Hong Kong: the Working Party, 1963).
12 Peter Hills and Anthony G. O. Yeh, "New Town Developments in Hong Kong," *Built Environment,* 9:3/4 (1983), 266–277. See also, Bristow, *Land-use Planning in Hong Kong,* 75–91.

13 Ibid.; see also Bristow, *Land-use Planning in Hong Kong*, 75–91; and W. T. Leung, "The new town programme," in T. N. Chiu and C. L. So eds., *A Geography of Hong Kong* (Hong Kong: Oxford University Press, 1983), 210–217.

14 Hills and Yeh, "New Town Developments," 266–277.

15 The number of reported industrial accidents rose from 34,405 in 1975 to 66,835 in 1979, with the death toll increasing from 212 to 301. See Cheung Wai-king, "Government policy towards employee benefits in the private sector: the case of workmen's compensation ordinance," M. Soc. Sc. thesis, University of Hong Kong (1981), 4.

16 Kuan, "Political stability and change in Hong Kong," 136.

17 Cheung, "Government policy towards employee benefits," 58–59.

18 Ibid. 54–70; and Queen Elizabeth Hospital comp., *Yiyuanre.qing.shi – Yilishabai yiyuan wushizhounian koushu lishi* ["QEH – A People's History. An oral history for the golden jubilee of Queen Elizabeth Hospital"] (Hong Kong: Cognizance Publishing, 2013), 11.

19 *Annual Departmental Report by the Director of Medical and Health Services for the Financial Year 1974–75* (Hong Kong: Governmental Printer, 975), 4.

20 "Urban services," and "Hygiene division" in *Annual Departmental Report by the Chairman, Urban Council and Director of Urban Services for the Financial Year 1961–62* (Hong Kong: W. F. C. Government Printer, 1962).

21 Hong Kong Urban Council, *The Urban Council, 1883–1983*, 23.

22 J. P. MacKenbach, "The epidemiologic transition theory," *Journal of Epidemiology and Community Health*, 48 (1994), 329.

23 David R. Phillips, "Epidemiological transition: implications for health and health care provision," *Geografiska Annaler. Series B. Human Geography*, 76:2 (1994), 75.

24 *Hong Kong Annual Departmental Report by the Director of Medical and Health Services for the Financial Year 1960–61; Financial Year 1965–66; Financial Year 1970–71; Financial Year 1975–76; and Financial Year 1985–86.*

25 *Hong Kong Annual Departmental Report by the Director of Medical and Health Services for the Financial Year 1975–76*, 1.

26 *Hong Kong Annual Departmental Report by the Director of Medical and Health Services for the Financial Year 1960–61; Financial Year 1965–66; Financial Year 1970–71; and Financial Year 1975–76;* and M. J. Colbourne, "Developments in medical education in Hong Kong in the Last 25 years," in G. H. Choa ed., *Recent Developments in Medical Education. Proceedings of the Seminar on Recent Developments in Medical Education held at the Chinese University of Hong Kong on July 6–7, 1978* (Hong Kong: Chinese University Press, 1980).

27 *Hong Kong Annual Departmental Report by the Director of Medical and Health Services for the Financial Year 1970–71*, 1.

28 *Hong Kong Annual Departmental Report by the Director of Medical and Health Services for the Financial Year 1960–61*, 36–37; and M. J. Colbourne, "Malaria in Hong Kong," *Society of Community Medicine Hong Kong Bulletin*, 9 (1978), 84–85.

29 *Hong Kong Annual Departmental Report by the Director of Medical and Health Services for the Financial Year 1970–71*, 8.

30 Starling et al., *Plague, SARS and the Story of Medicine in Hong Kong*, 23.

31 *Report on the Outbreak of Cholera in Hong Kong Covering the Period 11th August to 12th October, 1961* (Hong Kong: Government Press, 1961).

32 Ibid.

33 Starling et al., *Plague, SARS and the Story of Medicine in Hong Kong*, 45–48.

34 W. K. Chang, "National Influenza in Hong Kong, 1968," *Bulletin of the World Health Organization*, 41 (1969), 349–351; Starling et al., *Plague, SARS and the Story of Medicine in Hong Kong*, 54–57.

35 *Hong Kong Annual Departmental Report by the Director of Medical and Health Services for the Financial Year 1965–66*, 10.

36 *Hong Kong Annual Departmental Report by the Director of Medical and Health Services for the Financial Year 1975–76*, 3; *Financial Year 1978–79*, 3; and *Financial Year 1985–86*, 4.

37 *Hong Kong Annual Departmental Report by the Director of Medical and Health Services for the Financial Year 1965–66*, 14.

38 Starling et al., *Plague, SARS and the Story of Medicine in Hong Kong*, 238.

39 Ka-che Yip, "Health care in a harmonious society: crises and challenges in post-1978 China," in Joseph Tse-Hei Lee, Lida V. Nedilsky, and Siu-Keung Cheung eds., *China's Rise to Power: Conceptions of State Governance* (New York: Palgrave Macmillan, 2012), 190–191.

40 *Hong Kong Annual Departmental Report by Director of Medical and Health Services for the Financial Year 1983–84*, 4.

41 *Hong Kong Annual Departmental Report by the Director of Medical and Health Services for the Financial Year 1965–66*, 19; and *Financial Year 1983–84*, 9.

42 See chapter 7 for the discussion of the impact of the influx of Vietnamese boat people.

43 Steve Tsang, *A Modern History of Hong Kong* (London: I. B. Tauris, 2004), 205.

44 Wong, *The Political Economy of Health Care Development and Reforms in Hong Kong*, 83.

45 Xie Yong Guang, *Xianggang zhongyi yao shi hua* (History of Chinese medicine and pharmacology in Hong Kong) (Hong Kong: Sanlian Shudian, 1998); T. P. Lam, "Strengths and Weaknesses of Traditional Chinese Medicine and Western Medicine in the Eyes of Some Hong Kong Chinese," *Journal of Epidemiology and Community Health*, 55:10 (October 2001), 762–765.

46 Chak Kwan Chan, *Social Security Policy in Hong Kong: From British Colony to China's Special Administrative Region* (Lanham: Lexington Books, 2011).

47 *Development of Medical Services in Hong Kong, 1964*, 3.

48 Ibid., 30.

49 Ibid., 10.

50 Ibid., 19–20.

51 Ibid., 20, 23.

52 *Hong Kong Annual Departmental Report by the Director of Medical and Health Services for the Financial Year 1970–71*, 1–2, 47–48.

53 *The Future Development of Medical and Health Services in Hong Kong 1974*, 3.

54 *The Future Development of Medical and Health Services in Hong Kong 1974*.

55 Interview with Dr. Cai Xuanzhong, former Superintendent of Kowloon Hospital, April 6, 2013; Catherine Jones, *Promoting Prosperity: The Hong Kong Way of Social Policy* (Hong Kong: The Chinese University Press, 1990), 234–235. There was success, however, in the referral of patients from one hospital to another within the region. See Queen Elizabeth Hospital comp., *Yiyuanren.qing.shi*, 40.

56 *Hong Kong Annual Departmental Report by the Director of Medical and Health Services for the Financial Year 1983–1984*, 9.

57 Cindy Yik-yi Chu, *The Maryknoll Sisters in Hong Kong, 1921–1969* (New York: Palgrave Macmillan, 2004), 133.

58 Wong, *The Political Economy of Health Care Development, and Reforms in Hong Kong*, 83.

59 Timothy Man Kong Wong, "Institutional changes, research culture and professionalism: development of medical sciences in Hong Kong in the 1980s," *The Journal of Comparative Asian Development*, 7:2 (Fall 2008), 287.

60 Choh-Ming Li, "The new faculty of medicine of The Chinese University of Hong Kong: Opening Address," in G. H. Choa ed., *Recent Developments in Medical Education* (Hong Kong: The Chinese University Press, 1980).

61 Ka-che Yip, "Transition to decolonization: the search for a health policy in post-war Hong Kong, 1945–85," in Liping Bu and Ka-che Yip, *Public Health and*

National Reconstruction in Post-war Asia. International Influences, Local Transformations (New York: Routledge, 2015), 26.

62 *University and Polytechnic Grants Committee of Hong Kong. Report, July 1980 to December 1982*; and *Hong Kong Annual Departmental Report by the Director of Medical and Health Services for the Financial Year 1970–71*, 49.

63 *Hong Kong Annual Departmental Report by the Director of Medical and Health Services for the Financial Year 1970–71*, 50; and *Financial Year, 1983–84*, 16. Also, see Queen Elizabeth Hospital comp., *Yiyuanren.qing.shi*, 50–53.

64 *Hong Kong Annual Departmental Report by the Director of Medical and Health Services for the Financial Year 1983–84*, 1.

7 Diseases, socio-economic transformation, and transition to decolonization, 1980s–1997

Transition to decolonization

In a letter to the United Nations Special Committee on Colonization in March 1972, Huang Hua, the Chinese ambassador stated, "With regard to the question of Hong Kong and Macau, the Chinese government has consistently held that they should be settled in an appropriate way when conditions are ripe."[1] As the lease of the New Territories, negotiated in 1898, was due to expire in 1997, the status of Hong Kong became a critical issue that China and Britain would have to deal with soon in order to clarify the uncertainty of Hong Kong's political, and indeed economic, future. Conditions might be ripe for negotiation between China and Britain since the upgrading of Sino-British diplomatic relations to full ambassadorial level had begun at the beginning of 1971 and an agreement for the normalization of relations was reached just a few days after Huang Hua's statement. At that time, both China and Britain seemed to accept the continuation of Hong Kong's status quo during a period of unprecedented economic growth and expansion of social welfare services under Sir Murray MacLehose who became governor in November 1971. Yet toward the end of that decade, business interests in the colony were expressing concern regarding the approaching deadline of 1997 and its impact on the future of land leases and loan agreements as well as the overall economic development of Hong Kong.

Governor MacLehose's visit to Beijing and his meeting with Deng Xiaoping in March 1979 therefore assumed tremendous significance. MacLehose took the initiative to raise the "1997 question"; Deng reaffirmed China's sovereignty but assured investors to put their minds at ease. Talks between China and Britain began in 1982 and after two years of contentious and difficult negotiation, both sides initialed the Sino-British Joint Declaration in September 1984.[2] The Declaration stipulated that China would resume the exercise of sovereignty over Hong Kong beginning July 1, 1997. Based on Deng's "one country, two systems" formula, Hong Kong would become a Special Administrative Region (SAR) of China, enjoying a "high degree of autonomy," and maintaining the capitalist economic and trade system for 50 years after 1997.[3] Hong Kong's transition to decolonization had begun.

In order to understand how the Joint Declaration and subsequent Sino-British agreements affected socio-economic developments as well as policy formation and implementation in the 1980s and 1990s, we have to examine the key document that became the "mini constitution" of Hong Kong SAR (HKSAR), i.e. the Basic Law. The next step after the formal signing of the Joint Declaration in December was the drafting of a Basic Law of HKSAR by a committee in the National People's Congress of China. On April 28, 1988, the Draft Basic Law was published.[4] It was clear that Beijing wanted to retain final control over Hong Kong's political system, and the nature and degree of Hong Kong's autonomy in the future remained to be defined. Moreover, differences between the socialist legal system of China and Hong Kong's common law system had to be reconciled. However, the section on economy maintained that Hong Kong would be able to "continue to practice a low tax policy," to "practice free and open monetary and financial policies" and to maintain its "status...as an international financial hub." These provisions on economic development therefore reassured the business community that the capitalist system would continue and their investments and efforts to promote Hong Kong's economic prosperity would not be jeopardized; after all, any uncertainty or loss of confidence in Hong Kong's economic future would certainly impact the state of the economy and the allocation of resources to various sectors, including health and social services.

The Basic Law: health and social services

The Basic Law also contained specific stipulations regarding health and social policies. Essentially, HKSAR would be able to continue current policies or take new initiatives on its own. Articles 145 and 148 in fact dealt with three important aspects of Hong Kong's health policy: according to Article 145,

> The government of the Hong Kong Special Administrative Region shall promote the development of medical and health services and the development of Western and Chinese traditional medicine, and encourage community organizations and individuals to provide medical and health services of various kinds.

And Article 148 guaranteed that "religious organizations may, according to their previous practice, continue to run seminars and other schools, hospitals and welfare institutions and to provide social services."[5]

First, the inclusion of the development of traditional Chinese medicine (TCM) in the Basic Law was significant as TCM had been excluded from the colony's official health system and practitioners of TCM were not registered with the government. In China, however, TCM was recognized by the government, which, in fact actively promoted its research and encouraged the development of an "integrated" medicine that combined TCM and Western medicine.[6] As we shall see, TCM would indeed receive a new lease of life after 1997 and emerged as a recognized healing system in HKSAR.

Second, the Basic Law recognized the important role played by community organizations and NGOs in providing health care, in addition to public health facilities, for segments of the population, notably those who could not afford private care. The *kaifongs* and the many voluntary organizations that had been active at the grassroots would therefore be able to continue their work without direct interference from the HKSAR government. This would assure continuity of their work from the 1980s to the post-1997 period.

Third, the Basic Law guaranteed that religious organizations were allowed to continue their medical and social service work beyond 1997. It stipulated that the HKSAR government would not restrict religious activities that did not contravene the laws. Thus, religious organizations such as the Caritas should not have to worry that their medical and social service activities would encounter state opposition after 1997. In sum, the Basic Law made it clear that nothing would change as far as the provision of health care was concerned and the current health and social service policies in the 1980s and 1990s could essentially continue since there was no need to make adjustments based on speculations about the nature of government policies after 1997. Any modifications or changes during the 1980s and 1990s should be based on developments and perceived needs during that period. This was certainly welcome news to policy makers and officials who had been trying to devise a health care system that would hopefully provide, within governmental financial constraints, adequate support to those needing services. Still, throughout the 1980s and 1990s, as the demand for more government spending on all kinds of services grew, the government was always concerned about spending beyond its financial capability, and there seemed to be a fear of "incessant capital outflow" with the impending retrocession.[7]

Socio-economic developments: 1980s–1997

One scholar has argued that the watershed year for Hong Kong's economy was not 1997 but 1979, the year of China's opening and the launching of the "Four Modernizations" designed, among other things, to jump-start China's economy.[8] The "China factor," as we have seen, had always been a critical factor that affected Hong Kong's development, whether in population movements, economic growth, housing, or disease control and prevention. When the Joint Declaration was signed by China and Britain in 1984, some businesses had indeed adjusted to the new political environment by moving their registration out of Hong Kong or diversifying their assets in anticipation of 1997. The Tiananmen Square crisis in 1989 certainly helped to reinforce the feeling of foreboding that Hong Kong's political and economic future would suffer once it became part of China. Yet Deng Xiaoping's Southern Tour in January 1992 when he visited Shenzhen and Zhuhai to promote economic reforms and reaffirm China's opening reassured investors and the business community and helped to accelerate China's socialist modernization based on economic reforms that he had introduced earlier.[9]

The single most important feature of Hong Kong's economy during the 1980s and early 1990s was de-industrialization. Employment in the manufacturing sector as a percentage of total employment dropped from 41.3 percent to 12.3 percent in 2001, with only 400,952 workers remaining. The decline resulted in part from the exodus of capital to the mainland as labor-intensive processing and assembly plants were established to take advantage of the lower labor and land costs.[10] Hong Kong's investment in China rose steadily since the late 1970s and by the mid-1990s, Hong Kong accounted for the bulk of foreign investment in China, while China had also emerged as the second largest external investor in Hong Kong.[11] Moreover, the opening of China reinvigorated Hong Kong's entrepot trade as China's trade with other countries via Hong Kong steadily increased. In 1979, this entrepot trade accounted for 4.2 percent of China's trade; by 1996, it constituted 41.3 percent of China's trade.[12]

At the same time, a restructuring of Hong Kong's economy took place with the shift to financial and business services. By the early 1990s, Hong Kong had emerged as the global metropolis for Asia. The strength of its financial sectors and business services proved attractive to many international firms and it became the regional corporate management center for leading firms from North America and Europe. Hong Kong's ties with China certainly contributed to its success. The affirmation in the Basic Law that China intended to preserve Hong Kong as an international financial center helped to ease concerns of developments after 1997.[13]

Changes in the economy had adverse consequences, however, for many people, and, to a significant extent, affected their ability to get daily necessities and indeed access health services. The decline in employment in the manufacturing sector meant that a large number of manufacturing workers had to find jobs in other sectors; many of them ended up in low-paying positions in the service industries while many remaining in the manufacture sector received lower incomes. For the first time since 1985, the official unemployment rate of the city was above 3 percent.[14] In fact, research has shown that there was much inequality in income distribution among the population, and during the period 1994–1996, an estimated 600,000 people, or 10–15 percent of the population was living in poverty.[15]

The existence of substantial poverty was also evident among two social groups: immigrants from mainland China and the elderly. With increased cross-border travel and residence, Hong Kong-mainland marriages became common and the number of immigrants from the mainland rose in the 1980s and 1990s. Mainland China in fact became the major source of immigrants to Hong Kong, especially since the city had been accepting 150 persons per day from the Mainland to settle as permanent residents beginning from July 1995. By early 2013, Mainland Chinese immigrants constituted about 10 percent of Hong Kong's population.[16] For many of the immigrant families with children, adjusting to a totally different living environment often proved difficult especially when they oftentimes faced social exclusion. Many struggled in poverty as they could only secure low-paying jobs and lived on subsistence-level social security.[17]

The older people in Hong Kong also found themselves trying to cope with the problems of poor housing conditions, loneliness, depression, declining health, and general poverty. The fast growing aging population resulted from rising life expectancy and the decline in birth rate. In 1961, the aged 60 and above population constituted 4.8 percent of the total population; in 1991, it had increased to 12.6 percent.[18] Older people in Hong Kong were probably among the poorest in the population economically. Unlike those in government service or those working in private companies with retirement benefits, most retirees had to get by with their own savings or support from their family members.[19] A study of the aging population in 1979 actually claimed that 67,500 aged 60 and above residents lived in "sub-standard and often sub-human living conditions"![20]

Indeed, in the 1980s and 1990s, people in Hong Kong had to deal not only with rapid increases in expenditure on housing, but also on goods and miscellaneous services. One survey showed that by the late 1990s, recipients of the mean-tested Comprehensive Social Security Assistance Scheme spent about 58 percent of the per capita amount devoted to miscellaneous services and goods on medical services.[21] Certainly, these recipients could receive free medical services from the government, but that would mean long queues in public health facilities just to get an appointment and long waits – sometimes several years – for non life-threatening surgical procedures. Moreover, the government assistance scheme did not include coverage for consultation with TCM practitioners, nor for the purchase of proprietary Western and Chinese medicines for self-treatment if the individual chose to do so.[22] Not surprisingly, many elderly who often preferred TCM over Western medicine failed to find timely medical relief from mental health problems or diseases associated with aging if there were no intervention from community organizations or family members.

Cross-border health issues

The close cross-border link between Hong Kong and China in the 1980s and 1990s not only facilitated the flow of goods, people, and capital, but also led to heightened awareness of the many potential health issues resulting from the de facto creation of a regional production system as well as a common ecosystem. Certainly, Hong Kong had always been affected by developments across the border, but the opening of China and the huge increase in cross-border traffic and activities brought to the fore such issues as environmental pollution, sanitation, food safety, spread of pathogens, or risk behaviors practiced by travelers. The relocation of industry from Hong Kong across the border had resulted in the rapid and extensive urbanization and industrialization of the

Pearl River Valley. The lack of comprehensive environmental protection and control measures in the Mainland had created many environmental problems, including photochemical smog, contaminated water sources, pesticide and fertilizer overuse, and food contamination. These problems affected the health of Hong Kong residents directly as the city depended heavily on neighboring provinces for the supply of water and food. Many cases of food poisoning in Hong Kong during this period could be traced to imported vegetables contaminated with agricultural pesticides.[23] By the beginning of 1990, research showed that Deep Bay, a water body between Hong Kong and Shenzhen, had become the second most polluted body of water in Hong Kong after Victoria Harbor; deterioration of the water quality continued since 1990 as a result of pollutants pouring into the body of water from local livestock farms and "Shenzhen's sewerage and industrial waste."[24] The risk behaviors practiced by some cross-border travelers were also causes for alarm. The increase in truck traffic between Hong Kong and the Mainland and the behavior of some truck drivers facilitated the spread of sexually transmitted diseases. In fact, even during the SARS epidemic in 2003, a study revealed that travelers from the Mainland practiced less preventive measures such as wearing masks or washing hands.[25] Clearly, a regional approach based on cooperation and shared information between Hong Kong and neighboring provinces in the Mainland was needed. In 1988, the Hong Kong government and local authorities in Guangdong set up a system of inspection and registration of farms exporting foods to Hong Kong. Enforcement remained erratic, however, and some certified farms actually included produce from uncertified farms in their exports.[26]

Emerging infectious diseases

Hong Kong also faced a new set of challenges posed by the emergence of new infectious diseases in this period. The two most serious threats were HIV/ AIDS and avian influenza. How the government dealt with these threats highlighted the city's emergency preparedness for infectious diseases control, sector coordination, disease surveillance capability, and institutional support for those affected. Hong Kong's first AIDS case was confirmed in 1984 and China identified its first case the following year. In Hong Kong, sexual transmission had been the most important route of HIV spread, while only a small percentage of infections were due to drug injections. The government reacted quickly to control the situation, setting up an Advisory Committee on AIDS consisting of medical experts from the Medical and Health Department and universities to work out strategies to monitor the situation. The Medical and Health Department also established the necessary laboratory facilities and clinical expertise to screen, diagnose, and manage the disease. The following year, it formed a Scientific Working Group on AIDS to formulate and implement surveillance policies as well as medical and public health activities. Publicity and educational programs were introduced, based on guidelines of the World Health Organization, not only to alert and educate the public about the disease but also to urge voluntary reporting – a system put in place since 1985. Moreover, the Hong Kong Red Cross Transfusion Service initiated a program of blood screening to safeguard the supply of blood in August 1985.[27] Thanks to these efforts, the cumulative figures of HIV sufferers remained low: 957 from 1984 to 1997. And since the volume of cross-border traffic between Hong Kong and the Pearl River region remained extremely high (about 300,000 daily passengers) the government's HIV Surveillance Office cooperated with the cities in the region to share and update data on the HIV/AIDS situation. Many NGOs also undertook community programs on prevention: these included the Hong Kong AIDS Foundation and the Hong Kong Coalition of AIDS Service Organizations.[28] Yet, the level of discriminatory attitudes toward people with HIV/AIDS remained high, and as late as early 2015, the disease is still very much a taboo subject in Hong Kong and the stigma over AIDS remains the biggest obstacle in identifying and treating patients.[29] It is important, however, to note that Hong Kong's response to the HIV/AIDS threat was in many ways in sharp contrast to that in China where initially the disease was branded as a foreign disease associated with illicit behavior and little information on the disease was made public. It was only after the outbreak of the SARS epidemic in 2003 that a comprehensive program to deal with HIV/AIDS was developed.[30]

An emerging infectious disease that affected Hong Kong in 1997 before and after its return to China was avian influenza A (H5N1) that killed large numbers of poultry in chicken farms in April of that year. In May, a three-year old boy died from the first case of human infection with H5 virus, and by December, the total number of confirmed new cases rose to 17, of which five were fatal. Scientific studies revealed a direct chicken-to-human cross-species transmission of the virus had taken place without the involvement of an intermediate host. Thus, when poultry was determined to be the direct source of human influenza A and 20 percent of the chickens in the market were infected with the virus, the Hong Kong government took the drastic step on December 28, 1997 to cull all 1.5 million chickens in farms and markets in Hong Kong. At the same time, since a large portion of the live chickens consumed by Hong Kong residents were from China, all import of live poultry was temporarily suspended. Since there was no dedicated slaughtering facility in the city, all slaughtering of live poultry was done in retail markets and shops, and the possibility of the virus spreading was extremely high. Trade and sale of live poultry ceased for seven weeks so that all wet markets could conduct thorough cleansing. All these measures were a tremendous blow to the economy of Hong Kong's poultry industry, with its many chicken and duck farms. It also adversely affected the livelihood of poultry vendors and restaurant owners, not to mention the choices of consumers because of the prevailing culinary preference for freshly killed meat. These decisive actions, however, were instrumental in halting the further spread of the epidemic.[31] Hong Kong's success showed that at that time, with decisive and timely actions, the existing public health protection infrastructure, and the disease surveillance system were adequate enough to prevent a potential influenza pandemic. The crisis, however, had strained cross-border relations as China had rejected the suspicion that surfaced in 1998 that the H5N1 virus had originated in China,[32] and poultry producers in the Mainland also suffered financially when Hong Kong suspended all imports of live chickens. We shall examine in greater detail Hong Kong SAR's pandemic preparedness after December 1997 in dealing with outbreaks of H5N1 influenza in the next chapter.

Re-emerging infectious diseases

Emerging diseases such as HIV/AIDS and avian influenza were not the only public health challenges that Hong Kong had to confront during the 1980s and 1990s. Owing to a variety of reasons, such infectious diseases as malaria and cholera that had been under control for some time re-emerged and posed serious threats to the city's public health. As we have seen, a total interruption of local transmission of malaria had been achieved in 1969 and there was not one single indigenous case reported between 1969 and 1976. From 1976 onwards, except for a few indigenous cases, the bulk of the reported cases were imported, with the largest number occurring in the mid and late 1980s. In 1985, there were 161 imported cases; the figure rose to 741 in 1989.[33] Some of the cases in Sai Kung in the New Territories resulted from the continuous movement of people with low immunity against malaria into areas that were previously vector-infested. Hong Kong was, of course, vulnerable to imported diseases, especially from neighboring countries such as India, Pakistan, and Southeast Asian countries where malaria was endemic. Visitors as well as legal and illegal immigrants from China also contributed to the increased incidences of the disease in the 1980s. Thanks to the existing system of surveillance, investigation, and treatment as well as larviciding measures, the Medical and Health Department had been successful in monitoring and controlling the situation.[34] In 1985, following the recommendation of the WHO, a central reference laboratory for the identification of malaria was set up to coordinate the work of all government pathology institutes and laboratories.[35]

The most serious threat, however, was from the influx of Vietnamese boat people from the mid-1970s to the 1990s. In early May 1975, the first group of Vietnamese fleeing from their homes after the establishment of a communist government in Vietnam found their way to Hong Kong. The flood of boat people continued, abated by the Vietnamese government's ethnic cleansing policy that caused many ethnic Chinese to seek refuge in Hong Kong and elsewhere. The more than 200,000 Vietnamese refugees that arrived in Hong Kong during the late 1970s and 1980s were housed in various refugee camps while they were being processed and waited for resettlement in other countries.[36] Hong Kong's resources were severely strained and the government applied to the United Nations High Commission for Refugees (UNHCR) for material aid as well as requested the assistance of NGOs in providing medical and other services in the camps. In one of the camps, for example, medical services were provided by the Hong Kong Department of Health and two NGOs: the British Red Cross and the Save the Children Fund. A clinic took care of primary care, and notifiable diseases were reported to the Department of Health. At the same time, a disease surveillance system was set up to monitor any outbreak since the refugees originated from areas where infectious diseases such as malaria were endemic.[37] The spike of imported cases in 1989 – a total of 741 cases as compared to 97 in 1988 – resulted in a large part from outbreaks of the disease in two of the refugee camps in September and October of that year. The patients received treatment either in situ or in local hospitals and the Department of Health maintained that despite the continuing increase in cases, the situation was under control. At the same time, from September 1991 to January 1992, a measles epidemic among Vietnamese children occurred in one of the camps. The 16-week outbreak affected mostly children who were unvaccinated. In view of the spread of re-emerging infectious diseases, health authorities from Hong Kong, China, and Macau met in April 1990 to work out a regional monitoring and data exchange program to ensure better and more efficient sharing of information not only on malaria but also on other communicable diseases such as cholera, viral hepatitis, and AIDS.[38]

The high mobility of travelers in the region indeed dictated a regional approach to dealing with the spread of infectious diseases. The short but intense outbreak of cholera in Hong Kong in the summer of 1994 again proved this point. The last major cholera outbreaks were in the early 1960s and were part of the seventh cholera pandemic that spread from Indonesia in 1961. Since the 1970s, there were sporadic cases of cholera among tourists or Hong Kong residents becoming infected while traveling abroad. In 1989, a cluster of cholera cases occurred among 21 Vietnamese refugees in one of the refugee camps.[39] But in 1993 and 1994, there was a resurgence of cholera, with 30 reported cases in 1993, and a total of 50 cases in the summer of 1994, many of them imported. There had been outbreaks of cholera in the Lao People's Democratic Republic, Vietnam, and China in 1992 and 1993. At the same time, many cases were caused by the consumption of inadequately cooked or contaminated seafood. A common practice that helped to create the environment for contamination of seafood was the use of heavily polluted water in fish tanks in restaurants, or in fish-tank barges used for the transportation of fish. Hong Kong's coastal waters had been heavily polluted, and the risk of transmission was extremely high if polluted water was used directly in food preparation. The short but intense outbreak in summer 1994 prompted the government to regulate the bacteriological standard of water in fish tanks with the same standard set for seawater for swimming and other recreational purpose in public beaches. Moreover, the government intensified food surveillance at import, wholesale, and retail levels to ensure food safety, while health education campaigns were conducted to alert the public and travelers of ways to prevent cholera infection.[40]

Public health services

Hong Kong's success in controlling emerging and re-emerging infectious diseases owed much to the established public health infrastructure that had served the city since the 1970s; the Medical and Health Department had been able to respond quickly to public health threats and initiate new programs and necessary actions as in the case of HIV/AIDs and avian influenza. But with Hong Kong's status as an international financial hub and tourist site and the ensuring high volume of visitors entering the city at any given day, it became clear that Hong Kong remained extremely vulnerable to disease outbreaks in neighboring countries, and indeed, in other parts of the world. Increasingly, Hong Kong established partnerships with countries at regional and global levels as well as international agencies to promote prevention and preparedness, to monitor developments and disseminate information, and to cooperate in the containment of disease outbreaks. We have noted the increasing cooperation between Hong Kong and provincial governments in China. At the international level, Hong Kong worked, for example, closely with the Global Task Force on Cholera Control launched by the WHO in 1992 to coordinate activities of governments, NGOs and scientific institutions in combating epidemic enteric diseases and developing guidelines and training materials for cholera control. The WHO Regional Office for the Western Pacific also initiated a tri-partite surveillance program involving China, Hong Kong, and Macau.[41]

There were also structural changes in the provision of public health services in 1989. In 1985, the government released a commissioned report: *The Review of Delivery of Medical Services in Hospitals* (the Scott Report) as a follow-up study to the 1974 White Paper on the development of medical services in Hong Kong that had made recommendations for initiatives in the 10-year period after 1974. The Scott Report, however, focused only on the management of hospital services. The most important of its recommendations was the establishment of an independent hospital authority that would oversee all government and government-assisted hospitals.[42] We shall discuss in greater detail the nature and significance of the proposed hospital authority later in this chapter. With the projected establishment of the hospital authority, the former Medical and Health Department was reorganized into the Department of Health that became the government's "health advisor and agency to execute health care policies and statutory functions," and provided preventive, curative, and rehabilitative services to the community.

In its regulatory role, the Department continued to oversee the work of the Port Health Office that enforced both local and international health regulations to prevent the spread of communicable diseases. The work of the Port Health Office certainly took on added importance as Hong Kong assumed the status of a global city. The licensing and registration of health care institutions and personnel also fell under the jurisdiction of the Department. In its advisory role, the Department helped to formulate health policy and supported the work of other agencies and departments. Preventive services, as before, constituted an essential part of its responsibilities. These included maintaining surveillance, and conducting epidemiological investigations, of disease outbreaks; providing diagnostic and public health laboratory services; and playing a key role in the prevention and control of tuberculosis as well as operating a number of chest clinics offering out-patient services. Its Family Health Service provided antenatal and postnatal care, family planning, child assessment, and immunization against childhood diseases. The Department also continued its role in operating the Student Health Service that had its origin in the 1960s, and its duties ranged from physical examinations and health counseling of schoolchildren to referring students with medical problems to the care of appropriate medical providers.[43]

Public medical services

In addition to its essential preventive services, the Department of Health also had a role in providing some curative services to the population. In 1989, it operated 68 public out-patient clinics whose main duties were to identify and isolate communicable diseases, to screen acute from non-acute cases, and to treat minor ailments.[44] Yet they were not recognized as primary medical and health care providers – primary care was in fact mainly taken care of by the private sector. Critics had pointed out that the functions of these clinics should be enhanced or modified to provide primary care and not merely to serve as centers for screening, infectious disease surveillance, and serving patients with minor ailments. In fact, these clinics became increasingly less relevant as the disease profile of Hong Kong had, as noted, changed to the point where most of the morbidity and deaths were associated with chronic and malignant diseases.[45]

Certainly, the government had begun to pay more attention to curative care by the second half of the 1960s as the postwar heavy investment in public health and anti-communicable disease programs had succeeded in controlling or even eradicating some of the most common diseases. Yet, as we have seen, despite the rising prosperity as well as significant changes in demographics and socio-economic conditions, there were no clearly defined long-term health care goals except for the long-held twin objectives of promoting the general health of the community to ensure economic growth, and providing, within the constraints of the health budget, public medical care, especially for those that could not afford private care. Funds had been allocated for the construction of new hospitals, but little was done to improve the primary care system that remained largely in the private sector – hence the long queues and waiting time in Accident and Emergency (A & E) Departments of hospitals since access to public medical care was universal and available at minimal cost and many utilized A & E services for primary care purposes.

The reforms undertaken in the 1960s and 1970s, as recommended in the 1963 White Paper and the 1974 study, *The Further Development of Medical and Health Services in Hong Kong* had focused mainly on the expansion of the public hospital and clinic system. The 1974 study had recommended, and the government had indeed adopted, a regional approach to coordinate and administer medical and health services. Yet, as noted, only government and government-assisted hospitals, not private ones, were mandated to join the regionalization scheme, and the latter could also refuse to accept uniform bed-pricing policy. These recommendations revealed that the government had continued to narrowly focus on the management and organization of public hospitals and failed to take into consideration the broad perspective of the health sector as a whole.[46] The Scott Report was no exception. The most important initiative proposed by the report was the establishment of a "statutory Hospital authority...outside the Civil Service but largely funded by Government. It would report through its own Board, the chairman of which would be independent." According to the report, this structural change would bring the government and government-assisted hospitals "together more clearly and fully within an integrated structure accountable to Government." Moreover, as noted, it proposed that a separate body would handle public health matters.[47]

When the Hospital Authority (HA) was established in 1990, it took over control of 38 public hospitals and health care institutions. Under the HA, the public hospital sector expanded rapidly, and by the end of 2013, it oversaw 42 public hospitals and institutions with 27,400 beds.[48] Hospitals had developed into centers of medical technology, research, and learning, and had become extremely costly organizations. In fact, it has been pointed out that the costs of operating the hospitals had "spiraled out of control and out of all proportions to the cost of other public facilities."[49] There was also the problem of having adequate personnel to provide care and administer the hospitals as the private sector generally offered more attractive remuneration packages for medical personnel and there was a constant drain of doctors from the public to the private sector. Indeed, one of the basic flaws of the HA system was the failure to coordinate the development of the public sector with the private sector which had not grown much in the 1980s and 1990s. In 1990, the huge public hospital system had 89 percent of all the beds, while 70 percent of the primary care was provided by the private sector that continued to dominate the provision of primary care in the 1990s. At the same time, while more than half of the doctors worked in the private sector, they only had access to 11 percent of the hospital beds.[50] Certainly, the private sector charged more than public hospitals, but they offered more choices based on the patient's preferences, and less waiting time. The growth imbalance between the two sectors persisted and the fundamental problem of making medical care more readily available to the public remained unsolved.

Traditional Chinese medicine

The issue of the role that TCM should or could play in the provision of medical services in Hong Kong also received some scrutiny as 1997 approached. Article 138 of the Basic Law of HKSAR stipulated that the SAR government "shall, on its own, formulate policies to develop western and traditional Chinese medicine and to improve medical and health services." Practitioners of TCM in Hong Kong included herbalists, acupuncturists, and bonesetters, and they were in private practice; in 1989, it was estimated that there were several thousand Chinese medicine practitioners.[51] As noted, they were not recognized by the government and had no legal authority to issue death certificates and had no access to hospital beds for their patients. Moreover, they were denied the right to practice surgery, undertake treatment of eye diseases, to possess and use antibiotics, and use such medical technology as X-ray and inoculation. They were therefore excluded entirely from the official medical system and did not receive any financial support from the government. TCM was popular in Hong Kong, especially among the elderly, but many patients actually used TCM and Western medicine concurrently or when they felt that they needed additional help after having consulted practitioners of Western medicine. Already in the 1970s, there were supporters of TCM, including some physicians trained in Western medicine, who pushed for the standardization of training and practice of TCM as a first step in the legitimation of TCM.[52] Neither the 1963 White Paper nor the 1974 study on the future developments of medical services in Hong Kong included discussions of the role that doctors of TCM could play in the delivery of medical care. It was not until the 1980s with the impending retrocession of Hong Kong that the government decided to initiate a study to review the use and practice of TCM in Hong Kong and to recommend measures to promote the proper use and practice of TCM.[53]

In August 1989, the government appointed the Working Party on Chinese Medicine which submitted its report five years later. The Preparatory Committee on Chinese Medicine that was constituted as a result recommended the setting up of a statutory body to regulate the practice, use, and trading of Chinese medicine, the establishment of a system of accreditation and regulation that included registration, examination, and discipline of practitioners of TCM, and a system of registration, licensing, and labeling to regulate the manufacture, distribution, retail, and import and export of Chinese medicine. These recommendations were subsequently included in the Chinese Medicine Bill that was approved by the Legislative Council of HKSAR in February 1999.[54] The role of TCM as part of Hong Kong's health care system finally received formal recognition after the retrocession. We shall discuss in some detail the development of TCM after 1997 in the next chapter.

Medical manpower

Despite the founding of the Chinese University of Hong Kong Medical School, the shortage of doctors of Western medicine persisted. The University of Hong Kong Medical School and the Chinese University Medical School produced respectively 150 graduates and 70 graduates a year. Also, as noted, graduates from non-Commonwealth countries could be qualified to register by passing an examination and the completion of an 18-month externship, and an increasing number of medical graduates from China gained registration through this method. In 1988, the local list of the Hong Kong Medical Council which registers and regulates the medical profession showed a total number of 5,636 doctors (registered and provisionally registered), equivalent to approximately one doctor per thousand population.[55] These numbers did not include the several thousand practitioners of Chinese medicine who were in the private sector, however. The drain of doctors from the public to the private sector continued throughout the period as lower monetary compensation, poor working conditions, and few opportunities for promotion persisted in the public medical sector. Moreover, a large number of doctors emigrated to other countries, especially Canada and Australia, as 1997 and the transfer of sovereignty approached even though those countries did not recognize the doctors' training and experience. With the establishment of the Hospital Authority and the expansion of the public hospital and clinic system, the shortage of doctors created serious problems of staffing adequate medical personnel to provide care and administer the facilities.

The impending transfer of sovereignty in 1997 also played a role in the development of post-graduate medical training. Up to that time, post-graduate medical training was not available in Hong Kong, and doctors, who went overseas for specialty training could gain specialist status through passing examinations in the U.K. or Australia. But there was no official registry for doctors with specific specialties. The push among doctors to have a registry of its own gained momentum after the Joint Declaration and the publication of the Basic Law since Hong Kong could no longer rely on the UK to certify post-graduate training. In 1988, the working party commissioned by the government to study the issue recommended the establishment of an Academy of Medicine for post-graduate medical training that was finally established in 1993. Its official mission was to "maintain the standard of specialist training and specialist continuing medical education… and continuous professional development…in the territory." Beginning in 1997, it also maintained the Specialist Register.[56]

The nursing profession was also hard hit by the emigration of nursing personnel from Hong Kong during this period. In fact, countries such as the United States where there was a shortage of nurses had been recruiting in Hong Kong. In 1989, 1,103 or 9.8 percent of the government's nursing establishment left their positions.[57] As noted, there was no university nursing degree training; in 1995, the majority of nurses were trained in 10 training schools in nine public and one private hospital with a total annual intake of 1,368 students.[58] In 1990, the Hong Kong Polytechnic University began a full-time Bachelor of Science program in nursing, and the first Department of Nursing in an academic institution began in 1991 under the Faculty of Medicine at the Chinese University of Hong Kong. Hong Kong University also established a Department of Nursing Studies offering a four-year full-time Bachelor of Nursing program in 1995. The establishment of the Hospital Authority with its concern of cost-effectiveness and efficiency, emphasized management, and a position of nurse manager now assumed direct managerial responsibility for all activities within her/his units. At the same time, a new position of health care assistant was created to help qualified nurses to provide basic patient care. Despite the expansion and standardization of nursing education in academic institutions, the shortage of nursing personnel remained a serious problem in Hong Kong. The colonial legacy of nursing training in hospitals finally ended in 2003 when all hospital nursing schools were suspended.[59]

The signing of the Joint Declaration in 1984 marked the beginning of the transition to decolonization, and the impending sovereignty transfer in a little over a decade later had, in many ways, impacted the development of health policies in the 1980s and 1990s. In many ways, Hong Kong was beginning to plan for the time after 1997 when it became part of China, and health leaders had to assume control of the health system without intervention from London. Doctors and nurses, for example, would be licensed and overseen by their own respective councils in Hong Kong, and post-graduate training and certification would be done in Hong Kong. Despite initial reluctance on the part of the government, the Working Party on the study of TCM was appointed to evaluate the use and practice of TCM in the colony, although it would be after 1997 that TCM finally won its full legal status as part of HKSAR's health care system.

Moreover, the growing political and economic connections between Hong Kong and China not only helped to shape socio-economic changes in the colony but also impacted the way emerging and re-emerging communicable diseases would spread in the region, as well as create pressing cross-border health problems. And as Hong Kong became a global city, it became particularly vulnerable to diseases such as HIV/AIDS, avian influenza, drug resistant TB, malaria, and cholera that, if not controlled, could threaten the health of Hong Kong residents and even create conditions conductive to the emergence of a pandemic. Increasingly, Hong Kong's health policies included a regional component as the colony worked with health authorities in China and other countries as well as international bodies such as WHO to share data and set up a sound and effective disease surveillance system.

Yet as far as most public health services were concerned, the priorities and concerns from the past continued: family health and school health services, immunization of children, maintaining a clean water supply, supervision of sanitation in markets and eateries, etc. helped to keep Hong Kong a healthy place for its residents. As for public medical care, the government continued its rather haphazard approach in developing the curative medical care system, focusing almost entirely on the expansion of the public hospital and clinic system without taking a broad approach to coordinate the public and private sectors. The creation of the Hospital Authority that took over the operation of all government and government-assisted hospitals aggravated the imbalance in the health care system as a large private sector continued to operate in primary care; and before 1997, TCM practitioners constituted an important part of the care providers in the private sector.

What boded well for the post-1997 period was the stipulation in the Basic Law that guaranteed HKSAR's freedom and right to develop its own health care system. In the next chapter, we shall examine the public health and medical care system in the postcolonial state, and evaluate the colonial legacy as well as innovations and changes in the system.

Notes

1 Hungdah Chiu, "The 1984 Sino-British Settlement on Hong Kong: Problems and Analysis," in Hungdah Chiu ed., *Symposium on Hong Kong: 1997* (Baltimore: School of Law University of Maryland Occasional Papers/Reprints Series in Contemporary Asian Studies, No.3, 1985), 4.
2 Liu Shuyong, *Jianming Xianggang shi* [A Brief History of Hong Kong] (Hong Kong: Joint Publishing Co., 2009), 302–317.
3 "Joint Declaration of the Government of the United Kingdom of Great Britain and Northern Ireland and the Government of the People's Republic of China on the Question of Hong Kong," in Bill Knight ed., *Hong Kong: 1985* (Hong Kong: Government Publications Center, n.d.), 1–16.
4 "The Basic Law of the Hong Kong Special Administrative Region of the People's Republic of China," reprinted in Hungdah Chiu ed., *The Draft Basic Law of Hong Kong: Analysis and Documents* (Baltimore: University of Maryland School of Law, 1988), 117–143.
5 Ibid., Articles 145, 148.
6 Deng Tietao and Cheng Zhifan eds., *Zhongguo yixue tongshi. Xiandai juan* [A general history of medicine in China. Volume on the contemporary period] (Renmin weisheng chubanshe, 2000), 282–476.
7 Kwong-leung Tang, *Colonial State and Social Policy: Social Welfare Development in Hong Kong, 1842–1997* (Lanham: University Press of America,1998), 127.
8 Yun-Wing Sung, "The Hong Kong economy through the 1997 barrier," *Asian Survey*, 37:8 (August 1997), 705–719.
9 "Records of Comrade Deng Xiaoping's Shenzhen Tour," *Beijing Times*, January 18, 2002, from en.people.cn/200201/18/eng2002118_88932.shtml. Retrieved on May 20, 2015.
10 Hung Wong, "The quality of life of Hong Kong poor household in the 1990s: levels of expenditure, income security and poverty," *Social Indicators Research*, 71:1/3 (March 2005), 431.
11 Sung, "The Hong Kong economy through the 1997 barrier," 712.
12 Ibid., 709.
13 David Meyer, "Structural changes in the economy of Hong Kong since 1997," *The China Review*, 8:1 (Spring 2008), 7–29.
14 Wong, "The quality of life of Hong Kong poor household," 432.
15 Ibid., 411–412.
16 Stuart Lau, "Mainland Chinese migrants since 1997 now make up 10 pc. of Hong Kong population," *South China Morning Post*, March 21, 2013. See also Jianfa Shen, "Population and Migration Trends in Hong Kong," *Geography*, 82:3 (July 1997), 269–271.
17 Liu, *Jianming Xinaggang shi*, 392; Sung, "The Hong Kong economy through the 1997 barrier," 719; Kam-yee Law and Kim-ming Lee, "Citizenship, economy and social exclusion of mainland Chinese immigrants in Hong Kong," *Journal of*

102 *Transformation & transition to decolonization*

Contemporary Asia, 36:2 (2006), 217–242; and Zhao et al., "Income inequalities under economic restructuring in Hong Kong," 467–470.

18 Iris Chi, "Mental health of the old-old in Hong Kong," *Clinical Gerontologist*, 15:3 (1995), 31–44.

19 Nelson W. S. Chow, "Ageing in Hong Kong," in David R. Phillips ed., *Ageing in the Asia Pacific Region: Issues, Policies, and Future Trends* (London: Routledge, 2000), 160.

20 Liu, *Jianming Xianggang shi*, 392.

21 Wong, "The quality of life of Hog Kong poor household," 416.

22 Ibid., 416–418.

23 Lee Shiu Hung, "Public health issues in Hong Kong and China," *Journal of Epidemiology and Community Health*, 53:3 (March 1999), 130–131.

24 Yok-shiu F. Lee, "Tackling cross-border environmental problems in Hong Kong: initial responses and institutional constraints," *The China Quarterly*, 172 (December 2002), 989.

25 Lee, "Public health issues in Hong Kong and China," 130; Joseph T. F. Lau, Xilin Yang, H. Y. Tsui, and Ellie Pang, "SARS related preventive and risk behaviours practiced by Hong Kong-mainland China cross border travellers during the outbreak of the SARS epidemic in Hong Kong,"*Journal of Epidemiology and Community Health*, 58:12 (December, 2004), 988–996.

26 Kerrie L. MacPherson, "One public, two health systems: Hong Kong and China. Integration without convergence," *China Review*, 8:1 (Spring 2008), 94–95.

27 *Hong Kong Annual Departmental Report by Director of Medical and Health Services for the Financial Year 1985–1986*, 3; and Oi-chu Lin, William H. F. Kam, and Suk-yan Chan, "HIV/AIDS in Hong Kong. The emergence and impact of an epidemic," in Yichen Lu and Max Essex eds., *AIDS in Asia* (New York: Springer, 2004), 145–151.

28 See the Hong Kong government's website on AIDS at www.info.gov.hk/aids/english.

29 Joseph T. F. Lau, H. Y. Tsui, and M. Phil, "Surveillance of discriminatory attitudes toward people living with HIV/AIDS among the general public in Hong Kong from 1994 to 2000," *Disability and Rehabilitation*, 25:24 (2003), 1354–1360; and Jeanette Wang, "HIV/Aids still largely a taboo subject in Hong Kong and much of East Asia," *South China Morning Post*, March 23, 2015.

30 Joan Kaufman, "Infectious disease challenges in China," in Charles W. Freeman III ed., *China's Capacity to Manage Infectious Diseases. Global Implications* (Washington, D.C.: Center for Strategic and International Studies, 2009), 3–14.

31 Paul K. S. Chan, "Outbreak of avian influenza A (H5N1) virus infection in Hong Kong in 1997," *Clinical Infectious Diseases*, 34 (Supplement 2) (2002), 558–564; and Renee Snacken et al., "The next influenza pandemic: lessons from Hong Kong, 1997," *Emerging Infectious Diseases*, 5:2 (March–April 1999), 195–203.

32 World Health Organization, "H5N1 avian influenza: Timeline of major events," from www.who.int/influenza/human_animal_interface/H5N1_avian_influenza_update.pdf. Retrieved on May 20, 2015; and L. D. Sims et al., "Avian influenza in Hong Kong, 1997–2002," *Avian Diseases*, 47, Special Issue. *Proceedings of the Fifth International Symposium on Avian Influenza* (2003), 832–838.

33 The Department of Health, "Statistics of infectious diseases in Hong Kong," *Topical Health Report*, 2 (2002), 27–28.

34 Danny Lo, "Malaria stalks trail of tourists," *Hong Kong Standard*, April 8, 1985; Lee, "Malaria in Hong Kong," 7–17; and C. K. Li, "Epidemiology of malaria in the New Territories Region, Hong Kong (1975–1980)," *Journal of the Hong Kong Society of Community Medicine*, 12:2 (1981), 29–40.

35 "Reference laboratory for study of malaria," *Hong Kong Standard*, January 7, 1985.

36 "Hong Kong refugee camp 1975–2000" from www.refugeecamps.net/Hongkong. html. Retrieved on May 17, 2015; Kwok B. Chan and David Loveridge, "Refugees 'in transit': Vietnamese in a refugee camp in Hong Kong," *International Migration Review*, 21:3. Special Issue: Migration and Health (Autumn, 1987), 745–759; and Stephen Pattison, "Vietnamese migrants in Hong Kong," *In Defense of the Alien*, 15 (1992), 138–142.

37 W. R. J. Taylor, "Measles in Vietnamese refugee children in Hong Kong," *Epidemiology and Infection*, 122:3 (June 1999), 441–446.

38 "66 more cases of malaria confirmed," *Hong Kong Standard*, October 4, 1989; "Malaria cases sweep past 500," *Hong Kong Standard*, October 25, 1989; "Call for action against malaria," *South China Morning Post*, April 21, 1990; and Taylor, "Measles in Vietnamese refugee children in Hong Kong," 441–446.

39 Center for Health Protection, Scientific Committee on Enteric Infections and Foodborne Diseases, "Epidemiology, Prevention and Control of Cholera in Hong Kong" from www.chp.gov.hk/files/pdf/epidemiology_prevention_and_control_of_cholera_in_Hong_kong_r.pdf. Retrieved on May 20, 2015.

40 Ibid.; and S. H. Lee et al., "Resurgence of cholera in Hong Kong," *Epidemiology and Infection*, 117: 1 (August 1996), 43–49.

41 See WHO's website: who.int/cholera/task_force/background/en; and Lee et al., "Resurgence of cholera in Hong Kong," 48.

42 *Report on the Delivery of Medical Services in Hospitals* (Hong Kong: 1985).

43 "Hong Kong: the Facts, Department of Health" from www.gov.hk/en/about/abouthk/factsheets/docs/health_department.pdf. Retrieved on May 21, 2015.

44 Anthony Ng, "Medical and Health," in T. L. Tsim and Bernard H. K. Luk eds., *The Other Hong Kong Report 1989* (Hong Kong: The Chinese University Press, 1989), 194.

45 Anthony Ng, "Medical and Health," in Richard Y. C. Wong and Joseph Y. S. Cheng, *The Other Hong Kong Report 1990* (Hong Kong: The Chinese University Press, 1990), 410–412.

46 Robin Gauld and Derek Gould, *The Hong Kong Health Sector: Development and Change* (Hong Kong: Chinese University Press, 2002), 78–84.

47 *Report on the Delivery of Medical Services in Hospitals. Executive Overview*, 2–3.

48 Peter P. Yuen, "Medical and Health," in J. Y. S. Cheng, *The Other Hong Kong Report 1992* (Hong Kong: Chinese University Press, 1992), 279; and "Hong Kong: The Facts, Public Health," from www.gov.hk.en/about/abouthk/factsheets/docs/public_health.pdf. Retrieved on May 21, 2015.

49 Starling et al., *Plague, SARS, and the Story of Medicine in Hong Kong*, 77.

50 Ibid., 397–398; and Albert Lee, "The need for integrated primary health care to enhance the effectiveness of health services," *Asia-Pacific Journal of Public Health*, 15:1 (2003), 62–67.

51 Tsim and Luke eds., *The Other Hong Kong Report, 1989*, 204.

52 Rance P. L. Lee, "Health services system in Hong Kong: professional stratification in a modernizing society," *Inquiry*, 12:2 Supplement (June 1975), 51–62; Lam, "Strengths and weaknesses of Traditional Chinese Medicine and Western medicine in the eyes of some Hong Kong Chinese,"; and Wong Tze Wai et al., "Prevalence and determinants of the use of Traditional Chinese Medicine in Hong Kong," *Asia Pacific Journal of Public Health*, 8:3 (July 1995), 167–170.

53 Chinese Medicine Division, Hong Kong Government, "Development of Chinese Medicine in Hong Kong," from www.cmd.gov.hk/text/eng/development/development.html. Retrieved on June 1, 2015.

54 Ibid.

55 Tsim and Luk, *The Other Hong Kong Report, 1989*, 191.

56 www.hkam.org.hk/HKAMWEB/pages_1_90.html. Retrieved on June 2, 2015; andTsim and Luke, *The Other Hong Kong Report, 1989*, 193.

57 Wong and Cheng, *The Other Hong Kong Report, 1990,* 404.
58 Frances K. Y. Wong, "Health care reform and the transformation of nursing in Hong Kong," *Journal of Advanced Nursing,* 28:3 (September 1998), 473–482.
59 www.nursing.hku.hk/cms/en/about-school/history-a-milestones; www.sn.polyu.edu. hk/en/about_school/milestones/index.html; www.nur.cuhk.edu.hk/en/about-us/direc tor-s-message; retrieved on June 2, 2015; and Wong, "Health care reform and the transformation of nursing," 473–482; and Wong and Cheng, *The Other Hong Kong Report, 1990,* 404–405.

8 Combating Global Epidemics in the Postcolonial State, 1997–2003

On July 1, 1997, the crown colony of Hong Kong officially became the Hong Kong Special Administrative Region (HKSAR) of the People's Republic of China. In his first policy address to the Provisional Legislative Council on October 8, Chief Executive Tung Chee Hwa chose not to dwell on political issues; rather, he focused on some of the most serious social and economic challenges HKSAR inherited from the colonial government: housing, an aging population, health care, education, environmental problems, and a changing economy that, according to Tung, were "insidious threats which are taxing our courage and determination." He outlined plans for housing reforms, the establishment of elderly health centers and promotion of residential care, improvements in environmental planning, review of the health care system, a legislative framework to recognize and regulate the practice of Chinese medicine, and enhancement of basic education.[1] Although the colonial government had been proactive in initiating some reforms in housing and social welfare, yet in general, its policy approach in health care had been sporadic, incremental, and bereft of the broad perspective and long-term planning that would enable the government to confront such fundamental problems as changing demographics, financial sustainability, and fragmentation of care. On other issues such as Chinese medicine, the colonial government had refused to entertain its legitimization and promotion, and only belatedly commissioned a study to review the role and practice of Chinese medicine in Hong Kong. For Tung, the success in dealing with the most pressing livelihood problems would secure public support for the administration, and, as one Hong Kong academic put it, "win the hearts of the people through the improvement of services."[2] In order to gain legitimacy and establish a creditable record of accomplishments, the Tung administration would be interventionist in designing programs to meet the demands of the postcolonial state. At the same time, external forces and developments in the late 1990s and early 2000s would also affect the new government's attempt to fulfill its promise to "promote the well being of the people" of Hong Kong.[3]

Postcolonial socio-economic environment

From the handover to 2003, Hong Kong confronted numerous crises, economic and health-related, that significantly impacted socio-economic developments in the first years of Tung's administration, with far-reaching consequences for HKSAR's future. As discussed in Chapter 7, from March to December of 1997, a high-pathogenicity H5N1 avian influenza virus caused serious disease in both human and poultry, and the government had to destroy 1.5 million chickens in December 1997. Outbreaks of avian influenza occurred again in poultry in 2001 and 2002. Concurrent with the avian influenza epidemic, Hong Kong was subject to a series of external shocks, beginning with the Asian financial crisis triggered by the collapse of the Thai baht in July of 1997. The crisis spread to many of the economies of Southeast Asia and East Asia, and by the beginning of 1998, Hong Kong entered into an extended recession. Although the economy regained some of its strength in 2001 and 2002, a new shock in 2003 in the form of the outbreak of the Severe Acute Respiratory Syndrome (SARS) slowed down its recovery with a decline in the tourism industry and drop in consumer spending as people stayed home; it would take some time before HKSAR experienced real growth again. All these events had a tremendous and sometimes debilitating impact on Hong Kong's socio-economic developments as well as significant implications for the government's formulation and implementation of social and health policies designed to enhance the wellbeing of the people during this period.

Not surprisingly, the Asian financial crisis adversely affected people's livelihood the most as both the stock and property markets collapsed in late 1997. The real GDP growth rate recorded a negative growth of 5.5 percent in 1998 and unemployment rose from 2.2 percent in 1997 to a high of 6.2 percent in 1999. There were sharp drops of consumer prices and property prices fell nearly 40 percent in value during the third quarter of 1998. By then, Hong Kong was experiencing a deflationary recession with rising unemployment.[4] Although some Asian countries such as Korea, Malaysia, and Singapore gradually recovered in 1999, Hong Kong's recovery stalled as its economy was predominantly a service economy no longer driven by domestic exports. Rising unemployment aggravated the income inequality that had been increasing since the 1970s.[5] Research has shown a strong correlation between income inequality and inequity in health and health care.[6] In an attempt to ease the decline in property prices and make more housing units available, the government's new housing policy announced in mid-1999 would provide a new subsidy scheme to first-time home buyers.[7] Yet, low-income households still found it difficult to obtain public housing and continued to spend a large share of their income on rent, thereby further limiting their ability to access health services, especially in the private sector if they chose to do so.

As noted in Chapter 7, the growing aging population had been experiencing increasing hardship. Unfortunately, changing socio-economic conditions had also eroded the traditional extended-family support and care many of them had, or had expected to enjoy. One-person households increased steadily since the late 1990s, from 14.9 percent in 1996 to 16.5 percent in 2006, revealing the continuing but gradual disintegration of vertically integrated nuclear families living in the same households. What is particularly worrisome is that persons over 60 years old constituted about 40 percent of the single householders. This had serious implications for health care policy as research has shown that socially isolated and depressed persons, compared with those who were not, were four times more likely to have a heart attack.[8]

The Asian financial crisis and the government's response revealed that it was still operating with the underlying principle that "maintaining a small and efficient public sector is a crucial aspect of fiscal policy," and the allocation of resources to social welfare would remain low. Despite some efforts to subsidize the poverty class in housing, education, and health care, total public expenditures as a percentage of GDP remained under 20 percent in most years, and were far below those in many developed countries.[9]

Chronic diseases

The aging population was indeed a major issue that had critical implications for the government's planning for public health expenditure, as well as medical manpower and facilities needs. The percentage of the aged 65 and over population increased from 10 percent in mid-1996 to 11 percent in mid-2006, and was projected to reach 13 percent in mid-2016. At the same time, as the low birth rate persisted, the growth of the aged 65 or over group increased more rapidly than that of the overall population. The shrinking of the working population as a result of aging could, in the long run, lower the government's tax revenue. The aged 65 and over group, however, were more likely to require medical care and hospitalization, and utilized a larger share of public medical resources and funding. Statistical data of the Hospital Authority in fact suggested that the hospitalization rate of a person aged 65 or above was four times that of a person below that age. To meet the increased demand for medical care, the Hospital Authority estimated that in the two decades beginning in the 2010s, Hong Kong would need an additional 8,800 hospital beds in the public sector and hundreds more of health care workers.[10]

Since the mid-1960s, the proportion of mortality caused by non-communicable diseases had grown steadily. The mortality rate of infectious and parasitic diseases had decreased from 96.1 to 11.9 per 100,000 population between 1961 and 1998. In that same period, the mortality rate due to cancer rose sharply from 73.0 to 161.1 per 100,000 population. For the aged 65 and over group, the surge was even more pronounced, from 510.5 to 987.7 per 100,000 population; the other leading causes of deaths included endocrine, nutritional and metabolic immunity disorders, as well as disorders of the circulatory and respiratory systems. Compared to the five leading causes of death for the general population from 1988 to 1998 – malignant neoplasms, heart diseases, pneumonia, cerebrovascular disease, and injury and poisoning – it became clear that while chronic diseases were not confined to those aged 65 and over, the elderly segment of the population was most vulnerable to chronic diseases that generally required expensive long-term care, especially when chronic diseases were in many cases associated with degenerative functions of the elderly.[11]

Health services for people aged 65 and above, however, were far from adequate during the Tung administration. In 1999, the government maintained 18 elderly health centers where people of that age group could receive integrated health services, including health assessments, physical check-ups, curative treatment, and health education. There were also 18 visiting health teams to provide some basic care and to train caregivers for the elderly. Geriatric services were provided in all acute hospitals, and to promote "aging in place," the government tried to provide residential care services through a "continuum of care" in residential care homes. But the population of that age group totaled more than 700,000 that year![12] And in 2002, it was estimated that 29,000 elderly individuals were on waiting lists for government-funded nursing home beds, but many died during the average 21-month waiting period.[13] Undoubtedly, the escalating medical costs related to the growing number of elderly with chronic diseases was an urgent issue that the Tung Chee Hwa administration had to tackle in the post-1997 period.[14]

Environmental health

In addition to cancer and heart diseases, respiratory diseases had also become one of the leading causes of death in the 1990s. The proportionate mortality due to diseases of the respiratory system increased from 15.8 percent in 1981 to 18.7 percent in 1998, and the mortality rate per 100,000 population jumped from 75.8 to 91.4 in the same period. Not surprisingly, the rates were even more pronounced for people aged 65 years or over: 806.5 in 1981, 931.0 in 1996 and 854.2 in 1997.[15] Hong Kong's air quality had deteriorated since the late 1970s, and the poor street-level air quality was particularly detrimental to people's health as this was the air being breathed. The high population density, the large number of vehicles, and the tall buildings that prevented air circulation all contributed to the health risk that people were exposed to daily. The decline in manufacturing had helped to reduce pollution of ambient air, but there was an increasing threat from the rapidly industrialized Pearl River region as pollutants from those industries impacted Hong Kong's air quality. Studies on diseases and air pollution in Hong Kong had shown that significant associations were found between mortalities for all respiratory diseases and ischaemic heart diseases, and the concentration of all pollutants when analyzed singly. Moreover, there were also significant associations between hospital admissions for all respiratory diseases, all cardiovascular diseases, chronic obstructive pulmonary diseases, and heart failure, and the concentration of pollutants such as nitrogen oxide, sulphur dioxide, ozone, and particulate matter.[16]

Founded in 1986, the Environmental Protection Department (EPD) coordinated and carried out pollution prevention and control activities, as well as promoting environmental audit, environmental management, and environmental reporting. From 1986 to the early 2000s, the government imposed license control over pollutant-producing industries and power plants. It also introduced programs to tighten vehicle fuel and emission standard. With the reorganization of the EPD in 2005, it also assumed the responsibility for environmental policy making.[17]

Air quality, however, was not the only concern of the EPD. It was also responsible for monitoring water quality and pollution as well as for planning and development of waste treatment and disposable facilities. Hong Kong's coastal water was highly polluted by untreated domestic sewage and industrial effluents. Agricultural wastes contributed to the degradation of water quality in most enclosed bays. The generally polluted waters raised grave concerns about contaminated seafood and the safety of bathing beach water quality.[18] In 1997, it had been estimated that 20 percent of Hong Kong oysters had Hepatitis A virus, and an average cadmium concentration exceeding the standard by 40 percent.[19] To enhance the sewage disposal infrastructure, the government expanded the deep tunnel collector system and treatment works that handle sewage generated from all districts around Victoria Harbor area. Additional expansion was planned for 2006. At the same time, the sewerage system was being extended to serve more rural village areas.[20]

Another serious concern was the quality of the drinking water that Hong Kong residents consumed every day. About 80 percent of the drinking water came from Dongjiang (East River) in Mainland China. In 2000–2001, studies of the river's water quality revealed that the lower section of the river was contaminated by organic and inorganic pollutants that had apparently found their way into Hong Kong reservoirs.[21] The EPD of Hong Kong and authorities in Guangdong Province had cooperated to improve the water quality through the removal of pollutants before they reached Hong Kong. Hong Kong and Shenzhen also worked together to implement programs to enhance the water quality of adjoining water bodies, including Deep Bay and Mirs Bay. Regional cooperation was not confined to the improvement of water quality; Hong Kong and mainland authorities also established a regional air quality monitoring network covering the entire Pearl River Delta in 2005 to gather and share data.[22]

Reforming the health care system

The above discussion has shown that the health of Hong Kong's population, like that in other developed countries, was very much affected by socio-economic and environmental factors. Lifestyle-related chronic degenerative diseases had been gaining in importance, and since these diseases affected mainly elderly people, they would continue to dominate the mortality statistics as the population aged. An International Monetary Fund/HKSAR study in 2005 estimated that old-age-related spending for households could increase by about 8 percentage points of GDP by 2030, and that public expenditure would rise significantly as early as 2015 if the existing health care system as well as its level of financing remained unchanged. The fiscal problem would be compounded by the shrinking of the working population, with the retirement of the elderly, and the lowering of the government's tax revenue.[23] To fulfill his pledge to reform the health care system, Chief Executive Tung Chee Hwa would need to formulate policies to deal with the fundamental problems of the system that he inherited: tackling the consequences of an aging population, financial sustainability, and the fragmentation of care.

Before 1997, there had been a number of proposed reforms of the health care system, including those recommended by the 1963 White Paper, the 1974 study: *The Further Development of Medical and Health Services in Hong Kong,* and the Scott Report of 1985. As we have seen, all the reports focused on the expansion of the public hospital and clinic system and did not pay adequate attention to the relationship between the public and private sector as well as to how public health services should be funded. The most far-reaching recommendation in the Scott Report had called for the establishment of a Hospital Authority to take over control of public and government-assisted hospitals and health care institutions, and a new Department of Health to assume responsibility over public health and general out-patient clinics. The Department of Health officially came into being in 1989, and the Hospital Authority in 1990. The public health sector had been operating under the guiding principle that "no one should be deprived of adequate medical treatment through lack of means," a premise that suggested the provision of public health care as a welfare service, and that only the needy would accept the long queues and waiting time for medical services in public medical institutions. However, since everyone can access the public medical system, this premise ignored the willingness of many who could afford to pay for services in the private sector, to seek help in public institutions because of the great differences in fees and improvements of the quality of medical care in the public sector since the 1990s. The public hospitals accounted for over 90 percent of the total in-patient admissions, while the Department of Health's primary care clinics took care of less than 20 percent of out-patient admissions. Primary care remained predominantly in the private sector and was woefully lacking. Even when it was available, many people delayed visits for primary care, and then when conditions that should have been taken care of by primary care doctors deteriorated, they visited the Accident and Emergency Department of overcrowded public hospitals. A working party report on primary care in 1989 had already criticized the system's emphasis on public hospitals and the neglect of primary care, as well as "the absence of a clearly defined and up-to-date overall health care policy."[24]

Another issue that the Tung administration had to deal with was the high cost of maintaining the public medical sector, especially in view of the growing elderly population and expected increase in medical costs. A 1993 document from the Secretary of Health and Welfare, *Towards Better Health* – the so-called *Rainbow Report* – had proposed various ways to increase public sector funding, including the charging of higher fees and insurance; but the proposal failed to win support from both the doctors and the public.[25] The first major study of the problem of costs and funding was the report, *Improving Hong Kong's Health Care System: Why and for Whom?* prepared in April 1999 by consultants from the Harvard School of Public Health, to assess the capability of the existing financing arrangement to meet future needs, and to develop some viable payment options.[26] While the report praised the health care system as relatively equitable, it criticized the variable quality of care, inefficient allocation of public resources, and the lack of viable means to maintain financial sustainability. It recommended a compulsory health insurance, as well as savings and insurance for long-term care. A most controversial proposal was the reorganization of the Hospital Authority together with the private medical sector into 12–18 Integrated Health Systems. The Hospital Authority's response to the report was revealing; it maintained that "changes in an evolutionary manner to the way our health care is financed and delivered would be more beneficial to the community than any revolutionary changes."[27] The Report indeed provoked much debate, but it was eventually shelved as there was little support for compulsory health insurance.

The issue of viable options to finance the health care system remained divisive and it was difficult to find one that would satisfy everyone. Voluntary insurance financed only a very small portion of health care costs, and general taxation and user fees had been the major sources for financing the health care system. Three years after the release of the Harvard report, the government issued another document entitled *Lifelong Investment in Health* that proposed new policies to tackle some of the long-standing problems. It indicated the government's interest in the development of an integrated health care service and better interaction between the public and private sectors. It also proposed a medical savings scheme called Health Protection Account. Under this plan, working persons reaching a certain age should contribute 1 to 2 percent of their earnings that would be used to pay for health services in public hospitals after the age of 65.[28] The financing recommendation failed to receive support from the public: low-income persons did not want more reductions in their take-home pay while other segments of the society expressed doubts about the quality and choices of services that they would get in return for higher contributions. The rejection of these post-1997 plans revealed that the majority of the people preferred to keep the tax-based financing system that had been in place since the colonial days, and that they were not willing or ready to alter radically the status quo. The future of the organization and financing of the health care system would receive another round of scrutiny after the SARS outbreak in 2003.

Chinese medicine

One of the outstanding issues that had been discussed before the retrocession was the role that Chinese medicine should and could play in the delivery of health care. In 1995, following the recommendation of the Working Party on Chinese Medicine, a Preparatory Committee on Chinese Medicine was appointed to prepare for the setting up of a statutory body and a regulatory framework for Chinese medicine. The Preparatory Committee submitted two reports in March 1997 and March 1999 respectively.[29] There was much political support from the HKSAR government for the professionalization and modernization of Chinese medicine, and supporters of Chinese medicine also believed that Hong Kong had the potential of becoming an international center for the study and research of Chinese medicine. In his 1997 policy address, Chief Executive Tung stated that "For the protection of public health, we aim to introduce a bill in the next legislative session to establish a statutory framework to recognize the professional status of traditional Chinese medicine practitioners; to assess their professional qualifications; to monitor their standards of practice; and to regulate the use, manufacture and sale of Chinese medicine."[30] The Basic Law had stipulated that the HKSAR could develop traditional Chinese medicine and Western medicine, and it would be up to the government to formulate policies to realize that objective.

In July 1999, the Chinese Medicine Ordinance was enacted, and the Chinese Medicine Council of Hong Kong was established to implement the recommendations submitted by the Preparatory Committee designed to regulate the practice, use and trading of Chinese medicine, as well the accreditation and regulation of Chinese medicine practitioners. Under the Chinese Medicine Council were the Chinese Medicine Practitioners Board and the Chinese Medicine Board; the former was responsible for the development and implementation of the regulatory system for Chinese medicine practitioners that included their registration, examination, discipline, and continuous professional training; the latter regulated Chinese medicines, including the licensing and regulation of Chinese medicine traders and registration of proprietary Chinese medicines, a process that included the testing and evaluation of their safety, efficacy, and quality. During the transitional period, those practitioners who were practicing Chinese medicine on or before January 3, 2000 could apply to become a listed Chinese medicine practitioner. They would be divided into different categories depending on their academic qualifications and experience; while some could register directly, others would have to undergo an assessment or take a licensing examination. The process to register Chinese medicine practitioners began in August 2000; by September 2006, 92 percent (i.e. 5,262) of registered practitioners were listed practitioners who gained registration under these arrangements.[31] And in 2001, the regulation of Chinese medicines, including the registration of proprietary Chinese medicines and licensing of manufacturers and traders in Chinese medicine began.

Academic training of practitioners of Chinese medicine at the tertiary level began in 1998 with the establishment of the first full-time five-year first-degree course on Chinese medicine at Hong Kong Baptist University. A year later, the Chinese University of Hong Kong also offered a four-year degree program. The students were placed in some Mainland institutions, local clinics, and non-teaching hospitals for clinical training. To train students aspiring to become a specialist in integrated medicine, the University of Hong Kong proposed to offer a combined program in Bachelor of Medicine/Bachelor of Surgery/Bachelor in Traditional Chinese Medicine in 2001/2002. At the same time, research centers were set up to conduct scientific study of Chinese medicines, develop new drugs and raise funds for research. The purpose of these education, training, and research programs was to "produce an adequate pool of high caliber professionals to support Hong Kong's development as an international center of Chinese medicine."[32]

The question as to how Chinese medicine would integrate into the existing public health care system was central to the promotion of Chinese medicine in postcolonial Hong Kong. The consultation document *Lifelong Investment in Health* released in 2000 had urged the Department of Health to support the work of the Chinese Medicine Council to regulate Chinese medicine, and to promote the exchange of ideas and expertise between Hong Kong and the Mainland. As a first step to introducing the provision of Chinese medicine in the public health care system, ways to set up out-patient Chinese medicine services need to be explored; at the same time, Chinese medicine should also be introduced in selected public hospitals. But models of interface between Chinese medicine and Western medicine had to be developed while the Chinese Medicine Council and the Medical Council of Hong Kong should explore areas of collaboration.[33] The progress in building a public Chinese medicine health care structure remained slow, however; many Chinese medicine clinics had been set up and operated by local universities and NGOs on a self-financing basis, but the plan to establish a public Chinese medicine clinic in each of the 18 districts of Hong Kong did not take shape until after 2003. These public clinics operated under a tripartite model involving the Hospital Authority, NGOs, and local universities, providing medical consultation for the local community.[34]

One of the major drawbacks of the training of Chinese medicine practitioners was the lack of a teaching hospital for graduates of Chinese medicine programs in local universities. In 2013, Professor Bian Zhaoxiang, director of the clinical division of Hong Kong Baptist University's School of Chinese Medicine, openly called for the building of such a hospital that "is needed to give Chinese medicine students a complete education, without having to spend their last year doing practicum in Guangzhou."[35] It was not until 2015 that the government reserved a site for the development of a Chinese medicine hospital and began a study of the actual mode of operation for the hospital.

The legalization and professionalization of Chinese medicine had helped to boost public confidence in Chinese medicine. In 2001, a government study found that Chinese medicine practitioners provided about 23 percent of all primary consultations; at the same time, another study showed that 23.6 percent of respondents utilized a combination of Chinese medicine and Western medicine.[36] What is interesting is that among Chinese medicine service users, middle-aged non-communicable disease patients were most likely to use both Chinese medicine and Western medicine out-patient services, while older patients without non-communicable diseases were more likely to use Chinese medicine as their main form of care.[37] With the increasing importance of non-communicable and chronic diseases, Chinese medicine could play a significant role in the postcolonial health care system. But Western medicine practice remained the dominant modality of patient care, and even though the government had taken steps to encourage interface and collaboration between Western medicine and Chinese medicine clinicians, few actual Chinese medicine referrals were made since the mode of collaboration had not been formalized within the health care system even by 2010, and there seemed to be inadequate understanding of the healing culture of Chinese medicine among Western medical doctors. The pattern of utilization of the healing modalities was a legacy of the colonial health policy that marginalized Chinese medicine and excluded it from the public health care system.[38]

Combating global epidemics

Although lifestyle-related chronic degenerative diseases dominated the post-1997 disease profile, yet as noted in Chapter 7, new or re-emerging infectious diseases continued to affect Hong Kong's efforts to create a healthy environment for its residents. Tuberculosis, including drug-resistant tuberculosis, remained a major problem. In 1999, it constituted 35 percent of the 19,847 cases of reported notifiable infectious diseases; in 2013, although the total number of cases had declined to 4,664, it still ranked second, after chickenpox, in the total number of notifications for notifiable infectious diseases.[39] The problem with avian influenza also persisted, despite the success in halting the spread of H5N1 avian influenza after the depopulation of chickens in December 1997. In April 1999, two cases of avian influenza A (H9N2) affecting humans were confirmed in Hong Kong for the first time, although the two patients recovered fully. But during 2001–2003, other outbreaks of avian influenza caused by H5N1 occurred in poultry and among wild migratory birds. The widespread re-emergence of the avian influenza viruses in 2003 and 2004 caused alarm and raised global public health concern owing to their effect on poultry populations, their potential to cause serious illness among humans, and their pandemic potential. In February 2003, a man died and his son fell critically ill after contracting avian influenza from their visit to the Mainland in January. Through vigilance in influenza surveillance in both human and animal populations, the situation in Hong Kong did not develope into a major public health threat. However, new outbreaks of avian influenza emerged by 2004 in Vietnam, Thailand, and other countries in Asia, including Indonesia, China, Japan, and South Korea.[40]

The effort to combat HIV/AIDS continued to focus on policies to prevent and control the spread of the disease. At the end of 1999, the cumulative total number of reported HIV and AIDS cases were 1,350 and 450 respectively, but by 2003, the respective figures had exceeded 2,200 and 650. About 200 new cases of HIV infection were reported each year. Sexual transmission was still the most common mode of spread of the infection, but infection among injection drug users was increasing as well.[41]

To formulate strategies for the post-1997 period, the Advisory Council on AIDS released a study in 1999: *AIDS Strategies for Hong Kong 1999–2001* that outlined the rationale for, and the framework of, new policies and strategies. The rising incidence of sexually transmitted diseases, the extensive cross-border travel between Hong Kong and the Mainland, the potential for the spread of infection among communities on both sides of the border, and scientific advancement regarding the treatment of the disease, were cited as the need for the formulation of new policies in the post-1997 period. The document stressed the importance of prevention and quality care that would include both medical treatment and psychological support. Community involvement, including cooperation with NGOs, would be necessary to develop and implement effective prevention and intervention programs, and to promote acceptance of people with HIV/AIDS. The Council advised against mandatory testing, and as had been the case, the public would be made aware of the benefits of testing through education campaigns. At the same time, the document called for the strengthening of the HIV surveillance system, and to expand the system to incorporate the surveillance and behavior monitoring of sexually transmitted diseases. Thus, except for the stress on the strengthening and widening of the surveillance system, the document did not offer any strikingly new approach to the containment of the diseases. Much still depended on voluntary compliance and initiatives on the part of individuals.[42]

Undoubtedly, Hong Kong remained a low HIV prevalence area although there was a gradual increase in the number of reports of HIV infection every year since the first case was reported in 1984. It was estimated that by 2004, there were about 3,000 people living with HIV in the HKSAR, and the prevalence in adult population was therefore estimated to be less than 0.1 percent as determined in surveys of different populations. The trend however, indicated that gay men were at the highest risk of contracting HIV. In fact, in 2013, the Department of Health announced that "record-breaking numbers" of HIV cases were recorded and the infection rate was highest among the men-having-sex-with-men community. It was however difficult to know if the reported figures reflected the actual situation as gay men might be less likely to come forward for testing because of the social and cultural stigma against homosexuality.[43]

The SARS epidemic

The emergence of SARS in 2003 was the most severe threat to the health of Hong Kong's citizenry, and the epidemic proved to be a defining event in the development of health policy in the short history of HKSAR. It exposed some of the critical shortcomings in the health care system, as well as the incompetence of, and lack of leadership among certain government officials; at the same time, it brought to the surface public discontent with the Tung administration as well as increasing wariness of the vulnerability of Hong Kong as a Special Administrative Region bordering Guangdong and South China, a likely center of new emerging viruses. The epidemic reached Hong Kong in March 2003, and it was not until June 23 that Hong Kong was removed from WHO's list of SARS affected areas. By then, the disease had affected 1,750 individuals, including 286 deaths.[44]

Beginning in November 2002, there was an intense outbreak of atypical pneumonia in nearby Guangdong province, and there was panic buying by people of certain Chinese herbs that allegedly could protect them. On February 11, the Chinese Ministry of Health sent a report of the outbreak to WHO which dispatched a team to Beijing on February 15, but they were not permitted to visit Guangdong. A doctor from Guangzhou, who had been treating patients with atypical pneumonia in a Guangzhou hospital visited Hong Kong and stayed in a hotel in Kowloon on February 21. The next day, the doctor, who was already unwell, was admitted to a local hospital where he later died. From this first index case, seven other people whose rooms were on the same floor of the hotel contracted SARS: three of them were from Singapore, one was from Vietnam, two were from Canada, and one was a local resident. These seven individuals subsequently transmitted the disease to Singapore, Vietnam, Canada, and elsewhere in Hong Kong. On March 4, the Hong Kong resident was admitted to Prince of Wales Hospital where he became the index patient of the SARS outbreak in the hospital, affecting over 100 medical and nursing personnel.

Toward the end of March, scientists at the University of Hong Kong had identified a new strain of coronavirus as the probable culprit of SARS. As SARS had spread into the community by the middle of the month, the government asked all students and school staff who had contact with SARS patients to stay home for one week, but many schools decided to close for two days at the end of March. On March 27, the government imposed new measures to combat the spread of the disease, invoking the powers under the Quarantine and Prevention and Disease Ordinance. Classes were suspended for all schools until April 6. People who had been in contact with SARS patients were to stay home for 10 days and reported for daily check-ups. All arriving passengers were required to fill out health declaration forms at all immigration border control points.

The epidemic reached its peak at the end of March and early April. At the end of March, 213 residents of Amoy Gardens, a housing estate, were hospitalized with suspected infection, with 107 of the total living in Block E of the estate. The entire block was placed in isolation while all residents were relocated to holiday camps on April 1 for a 10-day quarantine. Preliminary investigation suggested that the sewage and drainage system might have been involved in the spread of SARS cases in Block E.

Throughout April and early May, SARS continued to spread despite more stringent quarantine measures imposed by the government. By May, the disease had ultimately affected eight hospitals and more than 170 housing estates throughout the city, although the number of daily cases began to decline. For the first time since the outbreak, no new cases were recorded on May 24, a day after the WHO lifted travel advisory from Hong Kong and Guangdong. On June 23, the WHO removed Hong Kong from its list of SARS affected areas.

In terms of the public health measures taken by the government to combat the SARS outbreak, they were basically similar to control measures adopted in previous outbreaks or epidemics of infectious diseases: early detection notification, isolation, treatment, investigation, and control.[45] SARS was made a notifiable infectious disease once the first few cases of the disease were identified, and patients were isolated in hospitals while family or close contacts were placed under surveillance, initially at home, and later in isolation centers for 10 days. Investigation of the source of infection, tracing of contacts, disinfection of affected residences and buildings, and public education campaigns on personal hygiene were carried out. To protect Hong Kong from imported cases, incoming and outgoing travelers were screened for fever in addition to completion of health declaration forms.

Some of these measures proved to be difficult to implement, however. Since there was a lack of epidemiological information about SARS initially, control measures were often applied in a somewhat haphazard manner. Moreover, since there was no dedicated infectious disease hospital in Hong Kong, patients were admitted to general wards of various hospitals ill-equipped to handle the highly infectious disease, and outbreaks in hospitals involving medical staff and health personnel as well patients in the same ward exacerbated the situation. Without designated isolation centers for infectious diseases, contacts had to be housed in holiday camps or recreation centers to be quarantined. Failure to provide accurate and timely information relating to the epidemic from the government caused confusion, panic, and mistrust among the public. On March 14, Dr. Yeoh Eng-kiong, Secretary for Health, Welfare and Food flatly denied that SARS had spread to the community. But he had to admit several days later that there were in fact cases in the community after a professor of the Chinese University of Hong Kong contradicted him and informed the press that there were cases outside the medical community.[46]

Economic and political consequences

The SARS epidemic hit Hong Kong at a time when it was just beginning to recover from the Asian financial crisis. Business travel and the tourist industry in Hong Kong were severely impacted when the WHO issued a travel advisory in early April. Most affected were travel-related businesses and services, including hotels, airlines, and retail stores. Local consumer spending also dropped dramatically as people decided to stay home to avoid potential infection in the community. Fortunately, as the number of new cases declined by late April and early May, local consumer spending gradually picked up and attained once again the pre-outbreak level by the end of July. At the same time, exports and re-exports were apparently not affected as cross-border truck traffic data did not show any obvious decrease between March and September 2003. Economists generally agree that the negative economic impact on Hong Kong was short-lived, and once the epidemic ended and fear and panic subsided, the economy improved and continued its gradual recovery from the Asian financial crisis.[47]

The political impact of the SARS epidemic was far-reaching, however. Relations with the Mainland were to some extent adversely affected as many people in Hong Kong criticized the Mainland for covering up the severe nature of the outbreak in Guangdong, and for the lack of cooperation that hampered Hong Kong's anti-SARS effort. As early as late 2002, there were already reports of an outbreak of atypical pneumonia in Guangdong, but newspapers in the Mainland dismissed the appearance of an unknown virus as a rumor and repeated the government's position that there was no epidemic.[48] On January 23, health authorities in Guangdong produced an investigative report on the outbreak but neither Hong Kong nor the WHO received a copy. The relations between Hong Kong and the Mainland was governed by the "one country, two systems," policy under which Guangdong authorities had no power to communicate with their counterparts in Hong Kong, and the demarcation between Hong Kong and the rest of China was considered to be a territorial division. Only the central government in Beijing had the power to breach the division "even for the purpose of sharing information."[49] It was not until early April that Chinese authorities announced the number of SARS cases and deaths in Guangdong and gave the WHO investigation team permission to travel "immediately" to Guangdong.[50] The lack of transparency and cooperation on the part of Mainland authorities reinforced the perception among many that people died in Hong Kong because it lacked accurate and timely information on SARS and was therefore caught unprepared. Not surprisingly, the SARS epidemic deepened the suspicion and mistrust of the Mainland by many in Hong Kong who also blamed the Tung administration for the mishandling of the crisis.

To a significant extent, the mistrust of Beijing as a result of the SARS outbreak in Hong Kong spilled over to the debate over the proposed enactment of Article 23 of the Basic Law which instructed Hong Kong to "on its own" enact legislation against treason, secession, sedition, subversion, and theft of state secrets. There were already street protests against Article 23 in December 2002. One of the controversial items was the provision of a public interest defense for the press for publishing secret government information.

Beijing's tight control over, and censorship of the press regarding information on the SARS epidemic in China was viewed by many as contributing to the rapid spread of the SARS virus to Hong Kong and the rest of the world. The Tung administration was shocked by the huge turnout of over half a million people on July 1, 2003 on the streets of Hong Kong to protest the proposed enactment of Article 23 and to express dissatisfaction and anger over the mismanagement of the SARS epidemic, as well as the perceived incompetence of the Tung administration. The SARS crisis therefore revealed some of the tensions in the "one country, two systems" policy and highlighted a critical issue in the relationship between Hong Kong and the Mainland: what role could and should the press play in such an arrangement especially when critical information that was deemed "secret" by the Mainland authorities was essential to the safety and wellbeing of the people in Hong Kong?[51]

Reforming the health care system: lessons from the SARS epidemic

The SARS epidemic showed that with its current structure, the public health and health care delivery system in HKSAR was not able to contain expeditiously an unknown infectious disease that was different from previous infectious disease epidemics in its explosive spread, especially when it lacked a well-coordinated system of surveillance, investigation, treatment, and response, as well as contingency planning that would allow the various government departments and agencies at different levels to adjust rapidly to changing developments during the outbreak. Dr. Lee Shiu Hung of the Center for Health Education and Health Promotion at the Chinese University of Hong Kong, summed up succinctly the shortcomings of the existing system in handling such an infectious epidemic as SARS: "deficient communications between the Secretary (Ministry) level responsible for health policy and the management level responsible for operation of the hospitals...overcrowded wards, poor ventilation in some hospitals, lack of isolation facilities, inadequate intensive care facilities, staff already working under heavy pressure, difficulty in isolating and cohorting patients with suspected or possible SARS, particularly at the point of admission and immediately thereafter."[52] At the same time, the difficulties in getting accurate and timely information from the Mainland highlighted the urgent need to establish an ongoing mechanism to share and exchange information on infectious diseases between Hong Kong and Mainland authorities.

In May, the government set up a SARS Expert Committee to review the government's handling of the SARS crisis, and the capabilities of the health care system to manage epidemics such as SARS, as well as to make recommendations for improvements. The report, *SARS in Hong Kong: From Experience to Action* released at the beginning of October refrained from holding any specific individual responsible for the shortcomings of the government's response. It did point out some of the factors contributing to the health care system's problems in dealing with SARS at the early stages of the outbreak. These included poor communication between the Hospital Authority and the Department of Health; the absence of both a "comprehensive, multi-agency strategy for disease prevention and control that puts the health of the public first," and a contingency plan to deal with a major epidemic. Clarity in the command structure was lacking. Moreover, the report also faulted the absence of hospital outbreak plans that would have prevented or at least reduced the severity of the explosive spread of SARS among the medical personnel, hospital staffs and patients. Finally, the report pointed to one of the fundamental and long-standing flaws of the existing health care system: the weak interface between public and private sectors (including private hospitals, private laboratories, family medicine and traditional Chinese medical practitioners) that, in this case, hampered cooperation in surveillance of communicable diseases and infection control. The report urged closer cooperation with Mainland authorities on health matters. One of the most important recommendations was the creation of a "Center for Health Protection which would have the responsibility, authority and accountability for the prevention and control of communicable diseases."[53]

The government's conclusions, however, were challenged by the report of a select committee appointed by the legislature issued in July 2004. The report in fact singled out specific individuals for their respective failures in the handling of the epidemic. Dr. Yeoh Eng-kiong, the Secretary of Health, Welfare, and Food was censured for failing to provide accurate information to the public, and to properly monitor and supervise the Department of Health and the Hospital Authority; Dr. Margaret Chan, Director of Health, was criticized for failing to explore all avenues in seeking more information from the Mainland; and Dr. Leong Che-hung, Chairman of the Hospital Authority, was blamed for the failure to put in place adequate contingency plans to deal with a large outbreak of infectious diseases. Two days after the release of the report, both Dr. Yeoh and Dr. Leong resigned from their respective positions.

Following the recommendation of the SARS report, the Center for Health Protection (CHP) was created on June 1, 2004 to "achieve effective prevention and control of diseases in Hong Kong in collaboration with major local and international stakeholders." It coordinated and implemented measures to prevent and control diseases through real-time surveillance, rapid-intervention, research, epidemiology training, and contingency planning.[54] Moreover, closer cooperation with Guangdong and Macao on the exchange of information about infectious diseases was achieved through the establishment of an expert liaison group. Commenting a year after the SARS outbreak, the two chairs of the government's SARS expert committee stated that "we are in no doubt that Hong Kong is better prepared to combat any epidemic than it was one year ago."[55] Indeed, Hong Kong health authorities apparently had learned from their experience in the SARS outbreak. On May 1, 2009, within minutes after a Mexican traveler who had entered Hong Kong via Shanghai was confirmed as Asia's first swine flu case, police had cordoned off the hotel where the traveler had stayed, while more than 200 guests and hotel staff in the building were quarantined for a week. The patient was sent to a hospital that had been designated to handle swine flu cases. Officials put swine flu on the list of notifiable diseases, and residents were urged not to travel to Mexico. In mid-June, after 12 students at a local school contracted the virus, the government closed all primary schools, kindergarten, and special schools for two weeks. The quick action and imposition of tough measures reflected the health authorities' determination not to repeat the mistakes committed during the SARS epidemic.[56] Yet, as Dr. Lee Shiu Hung so aptly warned, "Hong Kong will continue to face the challenges of infectious disease, because of increasing environmental pollution, population movements, the influx of refugees and immigrants, the emergence of new infections, and the changing lifestyle and behavior of the population."[57]

Notes

1　www.policyaddress.gov.hk/pa97/english/light_e.htm. Retrieved on June 13, 2015.
2　Maggie Farley, "New Hong Kong chief stresses family issues," *Los Angeles Times*, July 2, 1997.
3　Anthony B. L. Cheung, "New interventionism in the making: interpreting state interventions in Hong Kong after the change of sovereignty," *Journal of Contemporary China*, 9:24 (2000), 291–30.
4　Hong Kong Institute of Economics and Business Strategy, *Asian Financial Crisis: Causes and Development* (Hong Kong: Institute of Economics and Business Strategy, University of Hong Kong, n.d.), 109–119; and Michael F. Martin, *CRS Report for Congress: Hong Kong. Ten Years After the Handover* (Washington, D.C.: Congressional Research Service, 2007).
5　Zhao et al., "Income inequalities under economic restructuring in Hong Kong," 442–473.
6　Hedley, "The role of public health in social justice: the next steps in Hong Kong," 121–122.
7　Hong Kong Institute of Economics and Business Strategy, *Asian Financial Crisis*, 114.
8　Grace Cheng, "Review of the health system," in Joseph Y. S. Cheng ed., *The Hong Kong Special Administrative Region in its First Decade* (Hong Kong: City University of Hong Kong Press, 2007), 768; and Iris Chi and Nelson Chow, "Housing and family care for the elderly in Hong Kong," *Ageing International*, 23:3–4 (Winter/Spring 1997), 65–77.
9　Zhao et al., "Income inequalities under economic restructuring in Hong Kong," 463–464.
10　*Hospital Authority Statistical Report, 1998/99, updated 2015*; and Richard M. F. Yuen, "The challenge of an ageing society from a health care perspective," *Public Administration and Policy: An Asia-Pacific Journal*, 17:1 (Spring 2014), 1–14.
11　*Hospital Authority Statistical Report, 1998/99, updated 2015.*
12　Ibid.; "Health care for the elderly," and "Care for the elderly," in *Hong Kong Yearbook, 1999.*
13　Gwen Taylor, "Hong Kong's health care reform: nursing an ailing health care system back to life," *Perspectives on Business and Economics*, 20 (2002), 8.
14　J. Woo et al., "An estimate of chronic disease burden and some economic consequences among the elderly Hong Kong population," *Journal of Epidemiology and Community Health*, 51 (1997), 486–489.
15　*Hospital Authority Statistical Report 1998/99, updated 2015.*

16 T. W. Wong et al., "Associations between daily mortalities from respiratory and cardiovascular diseases and air pollution in Hong Kong, China," *Occupational and Environmental Medicine*, 59:1 (2002), 30–35; and T. W. Wong et al., "Air pollution and hospital admissions for respiratory and cardiovascular diseases in Hong Kong," *Occupational and Environmental Medicine*, 56:10 (1999), 679–683.

17 "History and Structure, Environmental Protection Department" from www.epd. gov.hk/epd/english/about_epd/history/history.htm. Retrieved on June 25, 2015; and "Hong Kong: The Facts, Environmental Protection" from www.gov.hk/en/a bout/abouthk/factsheets/docs/encironmental_protection.pdf. Retrieved on June 25, 2015.

18 Brian Morton, "Pollution of coastal waters of Hong Kong," *Marine Pollution Bulletin*, 20:7 (July 1989), 310–318.

19 Grant O. Hutchings, "Hong Kong's environment – from pollution control to sustainability," *Perspectives on Business and Economics*, 20 (2002), 6.

20 "Hong Kong: The Facts, Environmental Protection."

21 K. C. Ho, Y. L. Chow, and J. T. S. Yau, "Chemical and microbiological qualities of the East River (Dongjiang) water, with particular reference to drinking water supply in Hong Kong," *Chemosphere*, 52:9 (September 2003), 1441–1450.

22 "Hong Kong: The Facts, Environmental Protection."

23 "International Monetary Fund, People's Republic of China – Hong Kong Special Administrative Region: Staff Report for the 2005 Article IV Consultation Discussions, January 6, 2006" from www.imf.org/external/pubs/ft/scr/2006/cr0650.pdf. Retrieved on June 25, 2015.

24 Cheng, "Review of the health system," 775.

25 Hong Kong Government, *Towards better health. A consultation document* (Hong Kong: Government Printer, 1993); and D. B Gould, "The reform of health care funding," *Hong Kong Medical Journal*, 7:2 (June 2001), 152.

26 Harvard Team, *Improving Hong Kong's Health Care System: Why and for Whom?* from fhb.gov.hk/en/press_and_publications/consultation/HCS.HTM. Retrieved on June 29, 2015; and *Hospital Authority's Submission on Improving Hong Kong's Health Care System, August 15, 1999.*

27 *Hospital Authority's Submission on Improving Hong Kong's Health Care System.*

28 Health and Welfare Bureau, *Lifelong Investment in Health: Consultation Document on Health Care System* (Hong Kong: Printing Department of the Government of the HKSAR, 2000).

29 Chinese Medicine Division, "Development of Chinese Medicine in Hong Kong" from www.cmd.gov.hk/text/eng/development/development/html. Retrieved on June 15, 2015.

30 Ibid.; For a discussion o the political process of the institutionalization of Chinese medicine after 1997, see Stephen W. K. Chiu, Lisanne S. F. Ko, and Rance P. L. Lee, "Decolonization and the movement for institutionalization of Chinese medicine in Hong Kong: a political process perspective," *Social Science and Medicine*, 61 (2005), 1045–1058.

31 See the homepage of the Chinese Medicine Council of Hong Kong: www.cmchk. org.hk/cmp/eng/#../../main_index.htm.

32 Chinese Medicine Division, "Development of Chinese Medicine in Hong Kong".

33 *Lifelong Investment in Health: Consultation Document on Health Care System.*

34 Food and Health Bureau, "Legislative Council Panel on Health Services, 2015 Policy Address" from www.fhb.gov.hk/en/committees/cmdc/extract_2015_4.html. Retrieved on June 30, 2015. An example of this type of collaboration was the Chinese Medicine Research Center set up in 2006 jointly by Queen Elizabeth Hospital, Hong Kong Baptist University, and the Hospital Authority at the hospital. See Queen Elizabeth Hospital comp., *Yiyuanren.qing.shi*, 237–239.

35 Linda Yeung, "Hong Kong urgently needs a hospital to teach traditional Chinese medicine," *South China Morning Post*, December 16, 2013.

36 The Hong Kong Polytechnic University, "Learning module 3 – Development of Traditional Chinese Medicine in Hong Kong" from chinesenursing.org/openaccess/sn378/module/module3b.html#. Retrieved on June 30, 2015.

37 V. C. Chung et al., "Age, chronic non-communicable disease and choice of traditional Chinese and western medicine outpatient services in a Chinese population," *BMC Health Services Research*, November 2009.

38 V. C. Chung et al., "Referral to and attitude towards traditional Chinese medicine amongst western medical doctors in postcolonial Hong Kong," *Social Science and Medicine*, 72: 2 (January 2001), 247–255.

39 *Hong Kong Yearbook, 1999*; and Center for Health Protection, "Number of notifications for notifiable infectious diseases in 2013" from www.chp.gov.hk/en/data/1/10/16/43/1429.html. Retrieved on June 30, 2015.

40 Sims et al., "Avian influenza in Hong Kong, 1997–2002," 832–838; Katharine M. Sturm-Ramirez et al., "Reemerging H5N1 influenza viruses in Hong Kong in 2002 are highly pathogenic to ducks," *Journal of Virology*, 78:9 (May 2004), 4892–4901; and Centers for Disease Control and Prevention, "Avian influenza A virus infections of humans" from www.cdc.gov/flu/avian/gen-info/avian-flu-humans.htm. Retrieved on June 30, 2015.

41 *Hong Kong Yearbook, 1999*; and *Hong Kong Yearbook 2003*.

42 The Advisory Council on AIDS, *AIDS Strategies for Hong Kong 1999–2001* from www.info.gov.hk/aids/acaannuals/annual98/strategy.pdf. Retrieved on July 1, 2015.

43 *Factsheet on HIV/AIDS Situation in Hong Kong (2004)* from www.info.gov.hk.aids.english.surveillance/sur_report/hiv_fc2004e.pdf. Retrieved on July 1, 2015; Christy Choi, "'Record-breaking numbers' of HIV cases recorded in Hong Kong as gay men still at highest risk," *South China Morning Post*, November 26, 2013; and Wang, "HIV/AIDS still largely a taboo subject in Hong Kong and much of East Asia."

44 The following account of the SARS outbreak is based on Lee Shiu-Hung, "The SARS epidemic in Hong Kong: what lessons have we learned?" *Journal of the Royal Society of Medicine*, 96:8 (August 2003), 374–378; and WHO, "Update 95 – SARS: Chronology of a serial killer" From www.who.int/crs/don/2003_07_04/en. Retrieved on July 1, 2015. The updated figures given by WHO of people affected in August 2003 showed a total of 1,755 people affected, including 300 deaths. See WHO, "Summary table of SARS cases by country, 1 November 2002–7 August 2003" from www.who.int/csr/sars/country/country2003_08_15.pdf?ua=1. Retrieved on July 2, 2015. The official account can be found in SARS Expert Committee, *SARS in Hong Kong: from Experience to action, Appendix III* (Hong Kong, 2003).

45 S. H. Lee, "The SARS epidemic in Hong Kong," *Journal of Epidemiology and Community Health*, 57 (2003), 652–654. See also Yip, "Segregation, isolation, and quarantine: protecting Hong Kong from diseases in the pre-war period," 93–116.

46 Loh and Civic Exchange, *At the Epicentre: Hong Kong and the SARS Outbreak*, xvii–xviii. For an eyewitness account of how the Queen Elizabeth Hospital handled the SARS crisis from the perspective of the medical personnel and staff, see Queen Elizabeth Hospital comp., *Yiyuanren.qing.shi,* 179–187.

47 Alan Siu and Y. C. Richard Wong, "Economic impact of SARS: the case of Hong Kong," *Asian Economic Papers*, 3:1 (2004), 62–83.

48 Congressional-Executive Commission on China, *Information Control and Self-Censorship in the PRC and the Spread of SARS* (Washington, D.C.: Congressional-Executive Commission on China, 2003).

49 Loh and Civic Exchange, *At the Epicentre*, 117.

50 World Health Organization, "Update 95 – SARS: Chronology of a serial killer."

51 Loh and Civic Exchange, *At the Epicentre*, 117–138. For additional discussions of the SARS epidemic and political participation in HKSAR, see Joseph Y. S. Cheng

ed., *New Trends of Political Participation in Hong Kong* (Hong Kong: City University of Hong Kong, 2014), 78–80.

52 Lee, "The SARS epidemic in Hong Kong: what lessons have we learned?" 374–378.

53 SARS Expert Committee, *SARS in Hong Kong: From Experience to Action*, October 2003 from www.sars-expertcom.gov.hk. Retrieved on July 8, 2015.

54 See the official website of the Center for Health Protection: www.chp.gov.hk/en.

55 Jane Perry, "Two Hong Kong politicians resign in wake of SARS report," *British Medical Journal*, 329:7458 (July 17, 2004), 130.

56 Center for Health Protection, "Swine and Seasonal Flu Monitor," 1:10 (November 26, 2009) from www.chp.gov.hk/flier/pdf/ssfm_26_11_09.pdf. Retrieved on July 27, 2015. Also, Vivian Wai-yin Kwok, "WHO set to announce flu pandemic," *Forbes*, June 11, 2009 from www.forbes.com/2009/06/11/swine-flu-who-pandemic-hong-kong.html. Retrieved on July 27, 2015.

57 Lee, "The SARS epidemic in Hong Kong: what lessons have we learned?" 374–378.

9   Conclusion

From a "barren rock" with an inhospitable environment and plagued by diseases, Hong Kong has evolved into one of the world cities with some of the best indicators of population health. In 2011, its infant mortality rate was 1.3 per 1,000 live births; life expectancy at birth for males was 80.5 years, and for females, 86.7 years.[1] These impressive figures, however, mask some of the serious problems in health care and disease control that Hong Kong faces: widespread environmental pollution, rising incidences of non-communicable diseases, an aging population and increasing chronic diseases, newly emergent diseases and the return of diseases once under control, inequities in access to health care, and income inequalities. Some of these problems are systematic, as in the case of underdeveloped primary care in the health care system; while others, as in the case of what the WHO labels "social determinants of health" that include high disparities in income as well as poor housing and environmental conditions,[2] point to the government's failure to address adequately issues of social welfare and urban livability. The way the government of Hong Kong is going to deal with these health issues will be influenced by its past experiences in building its health care system and the formulation and implementation of disease-control measures; at the same time, it will certainly need to devise new strategies to adjust to changing demands and realities.

This book has argued that past health policies and disease-control strategies in Hong Kong had been shaped, over time and at particular situations, by the interplay of such factors as state power and priorities, social dynamics and customs, cultural perceptions, an econometric approach to health, science and bio-political governance, as well as regional and international health developments. This is a necessary corrective to mono-causation explanations, whether they over-emphasize scientific breakthroughs that made it possible to target the causes of specific diseases, or attribute health policy formulation and implementation solely to the power of the state in imposing control through bio-governance. Such grand theories ignore the complexity of the intersections of all or some of the aforementioned factors that go into the formation of health policies. Some of the factors were more prominent at a particular time; as during the colonial period when British perceptions and assumptions of the filthy and unhealthy Chinese population dominated their early attempts to introduce measures to segregate and control the indigenes. In post-1997 Hong Kong, factors such as the new socio-economic and political environment, as well as the increasing impact of external factors such as pandemics of emergent diseases contributed to a more interventionist state in health care institutional reforms and disease-control strategies.

The year 1997 was not the Great Divide in the development of Hong Kong's health care system or policies to combat and control diseases. An econometric approach to health that encouraged strategies of prioritizing the growth and sustainability of the economy had underlay the British reluctance to invest heavily in public health reforms and infrastructural improvements throughout most of the colonial period. It had lagged in addressing the social determinants of health in order to improve the health of the population. The colonial government surely must bear the culpability in ignoring poor housing and environmental problems, especially in the Chinese community, partly because of its racial assumptions, and partly because of its econometric approach to health. Tung Chee Hua's pledge to improve the housing and environmental conditions in postcolonial Hong Kong have fallen short, partly because of resistance from vested interests, and partly because of the econometric concern for cost-effectiveness and financial sustainability, especially in attempts to improve the funding of the health system.

HKSAR inherited and continued the British model of having a public sector that provides hospitals and other types of care, and a minimally supervised private sector driven largely by market forces. Post-1997 Hong Kong also enlarged upon the principle that the needy would have access to health care, while simultaneously encouraging the institutionalization of private health insurance. The dominance of the public sector was perpetuated especially with the bourgeoning power and resources vested in the Hospital Authority beyond 1997, while the private sector continued to provide the majority of primary care services, thereby exacerbating the problem of imbalance between the two sectors that had its roots in the colonial period. This imbalance will continue to have a negative consequence for those who are sick but delay their visits to the fee-for-service primary care in the private sector, and are then sent to overcrowded public hospitals for conditions that should have been taken care of by primary care physicians.

Grassroots dynamics also remained a central element in the course of policy implementation, whether it was manifested in resistance, accommodation, or adoption. We have seen the resistance of the Chinese to what they viewed as intrusive and insensitive measures during the plague epidemic of 1894. During the SARS crisis in 2003, the mistrust of Beijing, engendered and deepened by its apparent lack of transparency, as well as the anger over the Hong Kong government's mishandling of the crisis, spilled over to the debate over, and public demonstration against, the proposed enactment of Article 23 of the Basic Law.

Just as people, commodities, and food can now move or be moved around the globe with unprecedented speed as a result of globalization, so can infectious diseases be transmitted globally as a result of the high volume and speed of human mobility. The prevention and control of emerging and re-emerging infectious diseases therefore depend more than ever on regional and international cooperation so that a global network of surveillance, monitoring, and research can be set up. Certainly, individual countries should at the same time work to develop a sound and effective system of health promotion and disease prevention. Hong Kong aspires to the development and maintenance of a first-rate health care and disease prevention system that could protect the health of its citizens. As a global city, however, Hong Kong cannot independently eliminate diseases that can spread with ease from, and to, other parts of the world. But it can certainly continue its efforts to improve its public health programs and health care system so that it will be ready to combat global pandemics as it has done in its struggle against avian flu, HIV/AIDS, and SARS.

Notes

1 WHO and Department of Health, Hong Kong, *Health Service Delivery Profile: Hong Kong (China)*, 2012.
2 WHO, "What are social determinants of health?" from www.who.int. Retrieved on August 15, 2015.

Bibliography

Abraham, Thomas. 2004. *Twenty-first Century Plague: The Story of SARS*. Hong Kong: Hong Kong University Press.

Airlie, Shiona. 1989. *Thistle and Bamboo: The Life and Times of Sir James Stewart Lockhart*. Hong Kong: Oxford University Press.

Ali, Harris S. and Roger Keil (eds.). 2008. *Networked Disease: Emerging Infections in the Global City*. Chichester, UK: Wiley-Blackwell.

Allan, W. G. 1973. "Tuberculosis in Hong Kong, ten years later." *Tubercle*, 54:3, pp. 236–246.

Anonymous. 2012. *Yanhe Yiyuan Lishi, 1922–2012* [History of the Hong Kong Sanatorium and Hospital, 1922–2012]. Hong Kong: Hong Kong Sanatorium and Hospital.

Bay, Alexander R. 2006. "The politics of disease: beriberi, barley, and medicine in modern Japan (1700–1939)." Ph.D. Thesis, Stanford University.

Benedict, Carol. 1996. *Bubonic Plague in Nineteenth Century China*. Stanford: Stanford University Press.

Bergère, Marie-Claire. 1986. *The Golden Age of the Chinese Bourgeoisie 1911–1937*. Trans. Janet Lloyd. Cambridge: Cambridge University Press.

Bonner, Thomas N. 1995. *Becoming a Physician: Medical Education in Britain, France, Germany and the United States, 1750–1945*. New York: Oxford University Press.

Bristow, Roger. 1984. *Land-use Planning in Hong Kong: History, Politics and Procedures*. Hong Kong: Oxford University Press.

British Parliamentary Papers: China. Vol. 24. 1971. *Correspondence, dispatches, reports, ordinances, memoranda and other papers relating to the affairs of Hong Kong, 1846–60*. Shannon: Irish University Press.

British Parliamentary Papers: China. Vol. 25. 1971. *Correspondence, dispatches, reports, returns memorials and other papers respecting the affairs of Hong Kong, 1862–81*. Shannon: Irish University Press.

Bruyn, George W. and Charles M. Poser. 2003. *The History of Tropical Neurology: Nutritional Disorders*. Canton, MA: Science History Publications.

Butters, Henry Robert. 1939. *Report on Labour and Labour Conditions in Hong Kong* (No. 8 of Sessional Papers for the year 1939).

Carpenter, Kenneth J. 2000. *Beriberi, White Rice, and Vitamin B: A Disease, A Cause, and A Cure*. Berkeley: University of California Press.

Chan, Chak Kwan. 2011. *Social Security Policy in Hong Kong: From British Colony to China's Special Administrative Region*. Lanham: Lexington Books.

Chan, Julia L. Y. and N. G. Patil. 2006. *Digby: A Remarkable Life*. Hong Kong: Hong Kong University Press.

Chan, Kwok B. and David Loveridge. 1987. "Refugees 'in transit': Vietnamese in a refugee camp in Hong Kong." *International Migration Review*, 21:3, pp. 745–759.

Chan, Lau Kit-ching. 1990. *China, Britain, and Hong Kong, 1895–1945*. Hong Kong: Chinese University Press.

Chan, Lau Kit-ching and Peter Cunich (ed.) 2002. *An Impossible Dream: Hong Kong University from Foundation to Re-establishment, 1910–1950*. New York: Oxford University Press.

Chan, Ming K. 1990. "Labour vs crown: aspects of society-state interactions in the Hong Kong labour movement before WWII." In Elizabeth Sinn (ed.) *Between East and West: Aspects of Social and Political Development in Hong Kong*. Hong Kong: Centre of Asian Studies, Hong Kong University, pp. 132–146.

Chan, Paul K. S. 2002. "Outbreak of avian influenza A (H5N1) virus infection in Hong Kong in 1997." *Clinical Infectious Diseases*, 34, pp. 558–564.

Chang, W. K. 1969. "National Influenza in Hong Kong." *Bulletin of the World Health Organization*, 41, pp. 349–351.

Cheng, Grace. 2007. "Review of the health system." In Joseph Y. S. Cheng (ed.) *The Hong Kong Special Administrative Region in its First Decade*. Hong Kong: City University of Hong Kong Press, pp. 763–825.

Cheng, Joseph Y. S. (ed.). 2014. *New Trends of Political Participation in Hong Kong*. Hong Kong: City University of Hong Kong.

Cheung, Anthony B. L. 2000. "New interventionism in the making: interpreting state interventions in Hong Kong after the change of sovereignty." *Journal of Contemporary China*, 9:24, pp. 291–308.

Cheung, Gary Ka-Wai. 2009. *Hong Kong's Watershed: The 1967 Riots*. Hong Kong: Hong Kong University Press.

Cheung, Wai-king. 1981. "Government policy towards employee benefits in the private sector: the case of workmen's compensation ordinance." M. Soc. S. Thesis, University of Hong Kong.

Chi, Iris. 1995. "Mental health of the old-old in Hong Kong." *Clinical Gerontologist*, 15:3, pp. 31–44.

Chi, Iris and Nelson Chow. 1997. "Housing and family care for the elderly in Hong Kong." *Ageing International*, 23:3–4, pp. 65–77.

Chiu, Hungdah. 1985. "The 1984 Sino-British settlement on Hong Kong: problems and analysis." In Hungdah Chiu (ed.) *Symposium on Hong Kong: 1997*. Baltimore: School of Law University of Maryland, pp. 1–17.

Chiu, Stephen, Lisanne S. F. Ko, and Rance P. L. Lee. 2005. "Decolonization and the movement for institutionalization of Chinese medicine in Hong Kong: a political process perspective." *Social Science and Medicine*, 61, pp. 1045–1058.

Chiu, T. N. 1973. *The Port of Hong Kong: A survey of its development*. Hong Kong: Hong Kong University Press.

Choa, Gerald H. (ed.). 1980. *Recent Developments in Medical Education*. Hong Kong: The Chinese University Press.

Choa, Gerald H. 1985. "A history of medicine in Hong Kong." In *Medical Directory of Hong Kong*. Hong Kong: The Federation of Medical Societies of Hong Kong, pp. 13–29.

Choa, Gerald H. 1993. "The Lawson diary: a record of the early phase of the Hong Kong bubonic plague 1894." *Journal of the Royal Asiatic Society Hong Kong Branch*, 33, pp. 129–145.

Choa, Gerald H. 1999. "Hong Kong's health and medical services." In Albert H. Yee (ed.) *Whither Hong Kong: China's Shadow or Visionary Gleam.* Lanham: University Press of America, pp. 153–186.

Choa, Gerald H. 2000. *The Life and Times of Sir Kai Ho Kai.* 2nd. Hong Kong: Hong Kong University Press.

Choi, Alex H. 1999. "State-business relations and industrial restructuring." In Tak-Wing Ngo, *Hong Kong's History: State and Society under Colonial Rule.* London: Routledge, pp. 141–161.

Choi, Christy. 2013. "Record-breaking numbers of HIV cases recorded in Hong Kong as gay men still at highest risk." *South China Morning Post,* November 26.

Chow, Nelson W. S. 2000. "Ageing in Hong Kong." In David R. Phillips (ed.) *Ageing in the Asia Pacific Region: Issues, Policies, and Future Trends.* London: Routledge, pp. 158–173.

Chu, Cindy Yik-yi. 2004. *The Maryknoll Sisters in Hong Kong, 1921–1969.* New York: Palgrave Macmillan.

Chung, V. C. *et al.* 2001. "Referral to and attitude towards traditional Chinese medicine amongst western medical doctors in postcolonial Hong Kong." *Social Science and Medicine,* 72:2, pp. 247–255.

Chung, V. C. et al. 2009. "Age, chronic non-communicable disease and choice of traditional Chinese and western medicine outpatient services in a Chinese population." *BMC Health Services Research,* November.

Colbourne, M. J. 1978. "Malaria in Hong Kong." *Society of Community Medicine Hong Kong Branch,* 9, pp. 81–93.

Colbourne, M. 1980. "Developments in medical education in Hong Kong in the last 25 years." In G. H. Choa (ed.) *Recent Developments in Medical Education. Proceedings of the Seminar on Recent Developments in Medical Education held at the Chinese University of Hong Kong on July 6–7, 1978.* Hong Kong: Chinese University Press, pp. 7–16.

Congressional-Executive Commission on China. 2003. *Information Control and Self-Censorship in the PRC and the Spread of SARS.* Washington, D.C.: Congressional-Executive Commission on China.

Cunich, Peter. 2012. *A History of the University of Hong Kong. Vol. 1, 1911–1945.* Hong Kong: Hong Kong University Press.

Cunningham, Andrew and Bridie Andrews (eds.). 1997. *Western Medicine and Contested Knowledge.* Manchester: Manchester University Press.

Cunningham, Andrew and Perry Williams (eds.). 2002. *The Laboratory Revolution in Medicine.* New York: Cambridge University Press.

Deng, Tietao and Cheng Zhifan (eds.). 2000. *Zhongguo yixue tongshi. Xiandai juan* [A general history of medicine in China. Volume on the contemporary period]. Beijing: Renmin weisheng chubanshe.

Digby, Kenelm H. 1922. "The objects of a medical society: an abstract of address delivered before the medical society in September 1919." *The Caduceus: Journal of the Hong Kong University Medical Society,* 1:1 (April 1922), pp. 20–21.

Dwyer, D. J. (ed.). 1971. *Asian Urbanization: A Hong Kong Casebook.* Hong Kong: Hong Kong University Press.

Echenberg, Myron. 2007. *Plague Ports: The Global Urban Impact of Bubonic Plague, 1894–1901.* New York: New York University Press.

Elvin, Mark and Liu Ts'ui-jung (ed.). 1995. *Sediments of Time: Environment and Society in Chinese History.* Taipei: Academia Sinica.

Emerson, Geoffrey C. 2009. *Hong Kong Internment 1942–1945: Life in the Japanese Civilian Camp at Stanley.* Hong Kong: Hong Kong University Press.

Endacott, G. B. 1973. *A History of Hong Kong*, 2nd ed., Hong Kong: Oxford University Press.

Endacott, G. 1978. *Hong Kong Eclipse.* Hong Kong: Hong Kong University Press.

Eng, Irene. 1997. "Flexible production in late industrialization: the case of Hong Kong." *Economic Geography*, 73:1, pp. 26–43.

Evans, Dafydd E. 1970. "Chinatown in Hong Kong: the beginnings of Taipingshan," *Journal of the Hong Kong Branch of the Royal Asiatic Society*, 10, pp. 68–78.

Evans, Dafydd E. 1987. *Constancy of Purpose: An Account of the Foundation and History of the Hong Kong College of Medicine and the Faculty of Medicine of the University of Hong Kong, 1887–1987.* Hong Kong: Hong Kong University Press.

Faure, David. 1990. "The rice trade in Hong Kong before the Second World War." In Elizabeth Sinn ed., *Between East and West: Aspects of Social and Political Devlopment in Hong Kong.* Hong Kong: Centre of Asian Studies, University of Hong Kong, pp. 216–225.

Faure, David. 2003. *A Documentary History of Hong Kong: Society.* Hong Kong: Hong Kong University Press.

Faure, David. 2005. "The common people in Hong Kong history: their livelihood and aspirations until the 1930s." In Lee Pui-tak ed., *Colonial Hong Kong and Modern China: Interaction and Reintegration.* Hong Kong: Hong Kong University Press, pp. 9–38.

Fenner, Frank. 1993. "Smallpox: emergence, global spread, and eradication." *History and Philosophy of the Life Sciences*, 15:3, pp. 397–420.

Fisher, Carney T. 1995. "The plague in Chinese history." In Mark Elvin and Liu Ts'ui-jung eds., *Sediments of Time: Environment and Society in Chinese History.* Taipei: Academia Sinica, pp. 673–745.

Garner, Jim. 1973. "The Lancet celebrates 150th anniversary, still following its founder's footsteps." *Canadian Medical Association Journal*, 109 (December 15), pp. 1254–1255.

Gauld, Robin and Derek Gould. 2002. *The Hong Kong Health Sector: Development and Change.* Hong Kong: The Chinese University Press.

Gibson, R. M. 1900. "Beriberi in Hong Kong, with special reference to the records of the Alice Memorial and Nethersole Hospitals and with notes on two years experience of the disease." M.D. Thesis, University of Edinburgh.

Gould, D. B. 2001. "The reform of health care funding." *Hong Kong Medical Journal*, 7:2 pp. 150–154.

Guan, Lixiong (Kwan Lai Hung). 1993. *Rizhan shiqi de Xianggang* [Hong Kong under Japanese Occupation]. Hong Kong: Joint Publishing Company.

Hambro, Edvard. 1955. *The Problem of Chinese Refugees in Hong Kong: Report Submitted to the United Nations High Commissioner for Refugees.* Leyden: A. W. Sijthoff.

Harrison, Mark. 2008. *Disease and the Modern World: 1500 to the Present Day.* Cambridge: Polity Press.

Hedley, Anthony. 2006. "The role of public health in social justice: the next steps in Hong Kong," In Gabriel M. Leung and John Bacon-Shone (eds.) *Hong Kong's Health Systems: Reflections, Perspectives and Visions.* Hong Kong: Hong Kong University Press, pp. 109–133.

Hills, Peter and Anthony G. O. Yeh. 1983. "New town developments in Hong Kong." *Built Environment*, 9:3/4, pp. 266–277.

Ho, K. C., Y. L.Chow, and J. T. S. Yau. 2003. "Chemical and microbiological qualities of the East River (Dongjiang) water, with particular reference to drinking water supply in Hong Kong." *Chemosphere*, 52:9, pp. 1441–1450.

Ho, Pui Yin. 2004. *The Administrative History of the Government Agencies, 1841–2002.* Hong Kong: Hong Kong University Press.

Hoe, Susanna and Derek Roebuck. 1999. *The Taking of Hong Kong: Charles and Clara Elliot in China Waters.* London: Curzon.

Hong Kong Anti-TB Association, 1960. *Annual Reports.* Hong Kong: Hong Kong Anti-Tuberculosis Association.

Hong Kong Council of Social Services. 1953. *Meeting the Social Challenge: A Survey of the Work of Voluntary and Government Social Service Organization in Hong Kong.* Hong Kong: Council of Social Services.

Hong Kong Department of Health. 2002. "Statistics of infectious diseases in Hong Kong." *Topical Health Report*, 2, pp. 27–28.

Hong Kong Government. *The Blue Book of the Hong Kong Government.* Various years. Hong Kong: Hong Kong Government.

Hong Kong Government. *The Colonial Surgeon's Report.* Various years. Hong Kong: Hong Kong Government.

Hong Kong Government. *Medical and Sanitary Reports.* Various years. Hong Kong: Hong Kong Government.

Hong Kong Government. *The Hong Kong Administrative Report.* Various years. Hong Kong: Hong Kong Government.

Hong Kong Government. *Hong Kong Annual Departmental Report by the Director of Medical and Health Services.* Various years. Hong Kong: Hong Kong Government.

Hong Kong Government. 1857. "Ordinance 12 of 1857." *Hong Kong Government Gazette*, 28 November.Hong Kong: Hong Kong Government.

Hong Kong Government. 1888. "An ordinance for reservation of a European District in the City of Victoria (amended)," 21 April, pp. 375–376. Hong Kong: Hong Kong Government.

Hong Kong Government. 1895. "Medical report on the epidemic of bubonic plague in 1894." *Hong Kong Legislative Council Sessional Papers*, 2 March 1895. Hong Kong: Hong Kong Government.

Hong Kong Government. 1896. "Minutes of Proceedings of the Legislative Council." *The Hong Kong Hansard.* 3 December.Hong Kong: Hong Kong Government.

Hong Kong Government. 1911. *Historical and Statistical Abstract of the Colony of Hong Kong.* 2nd. Historical Part. Hong Kong: Hong Kong Government.

Hong Kong Government. 1921. *Report of the Census of the Colony for 1921* (No. 15 of Sessional Paper for the Year of 1921). Hong Kong: Hong Kong Government.

Hong Kong Government. 1923. *Report of the Housing Commission* (No. 10 of Sessional Paper for the Year of 1923). Hong Kong: Hong Kong Government.

Hong Kong Government. 1938. *Report of the Housing Commission* (No. 12 of Sessional Paper for the Year of 1938). Hong Kong: Hong Kong Government.

Hong Kong Government. *Hong Kong Annual Report, 1950–51; 1952.* Hong Kong: Hong Kong Government.

Hong Kong Government. 1961. *Report on the Outbreak of Cholera in Hong Kong Covering the Period 11th August to 12th October, 1961.* Hong Kong: Government Printer.

Hong Kong Government. 1964. *Development of Medical Services in Hong Kong.* Hong Kong: Government Printer.

Hong Kong Government. 1967. *Kowloon Disturbances 1966: Report of Commission of Inquiry.* Hong Kong: Government Printer.

Hong Kong Government. 1968. *Hong Kong Disturbances 1967.* Hong Kong: Government Printer.

Hong Kong Government. 1974. *The Future Development of Medical and Health Services in Hong Kong.* Hong Kong: Hong Kong Government.

Hong Kong Government. 1985. *Report on the Delivery of Medical Services in Hospitals.* Hong Kong: Hong Kong Government.

Hong Kong Government. 1993. *Towards Better Health. A Consultation Document.* Hong Kong: Hong Kong Government.

Hong Kong Government. 1999. *Improving Hong Kong's Health Care System: Why and for Whom?*Hong Kong: Hong Kong Government.

Hong Kong Government. 2000. *Lifelong Investment in Health: Consultation Document on Health Care System.* Hong Kong: Hong Kong Government.

Hong Kong Government. 2004. *HIV/AIDS Situation in Hong Kong (2004).* Hong Kong: Hong Kong Government.

Hong Kong Government. 2015. *Hong Kong Fact Sheets – Water, Power, Gas Supplies.* Hong Kong: Hong Kong Government.

Hong Kong Government. 2015. *Chinese Medicine Division. Development of Chinese Medicine in Hong Kong.* Hong Kong: Hong Kong Government.

Hong Kong Government. 2015. *History and Structure, Environmental Protection Department.* Hong Kong: Hong Kong Government.

Hong Kong Hospital Authority. 1999. *Hospital Authority's Submission on Improving Hong Kong's Health Care System.* August 15. Hong Kong: Hong Kong Government.

Hong Kong Hospital Authority. 2015. *Hospital Authority Statistical Report, 1998/99, updated 2015.* Hong Kong: Hong Kong Government.

Hong Kong Institute of Economics and Business Strategy. 2000 n.d. *Asian Financial Crisis: Causes and Development.* Hong Kong: Institute of Economics and Business Strategy, University of Hong Kong.

Hong Kong Urban Council. 1962. *Annual Departmental Report by the Chairman, Urban Council and Director of Urban Services for the Financial Year 1961–62.* Hong Kong: W. F. C. Government Printer.

Hong Kong Urban Council. 1983. *The Urban Council, 1883–1983.* Hong Kong: The Urban Council.

Hong Kong Yearbook. 2003. Hong Kong: Hong Kong Government.

Hu, Yueh. 1962. "The problem of Hong Kong refugees." *Asian Survey*, 2:1, pp. 28–37.

Huang, Yasheng. 1997. "The economic and political integration of Hong Kong: implications for government-business relations." In Warren Cohen and Li Zhao (eds.) *Hong Kong Under Chinese Rule. The Economic and Political Implications of Reversion.* Cambridge: Cambridge University Press, pp. 96–113.

Hui, Po Keung. 1999. "Comprador politics and middlemen capitalism." In Ngo Tak-wing ed., *Hong Kong's History: State and Society under Colonial Rule.* London: Routledge.

Hunter, William. 1904. *A Research into the Epidemic and Epizootic Plague.* Hong Kong: Hong Kong Government.

Hunter, William and Wilfred Koch. 1906. *A Research into the Etiology of Beriberi, together with a Report on the outbreak in the Po Leung Kuk.* Hong Kong: Hong Kong Government

Hutcheon, Robin. 1999. *Bedside Manner: Hospital and Health Care in Hong Kong*. Hong Kong: The Chinese University Press.

Hutchings, Grant O. 2002. "Hong Kong's environment – from pollution control to sustainability." *Perspectives on Business and Economics*, 20, pp. 1–18.

"Inauguration of the Medical College: Public Meeting in Hong Kong – The Inaugural Addresses." 1887. *China Mail*, October 1.

Jarman, R. I. (ed.). 1996. *Hong Kong Annual Administration Reports*, Vols. 1–6. London: Archive Editions.

Jefferson, A. J. 1950. "A case of pernicious beri-beri." *British Medical Journal* (May 14, 1898), p. 1257.

Johnson, Sheila K. 1966. "Hong Kong's resettled squatters: a statistical analysis." *Asian Survey*, 6:11, November, pp. 643–656.

"Joint Declaration of the Government of the United Kingdom of Great Britain and Northern Ireland and the Government of the People's Republic of China on the Question of Hong Kong, 1984." 1985, in Bill Knight (ed.) *Hong Kong: 1985*. Hong Kong: Government Publications Center, pp. 1–16.

Jones, Catherine M. 1990. *Promoting Prosperity: The Hong Kong Way of Social Policy*. Hong Kong: The Chinese University Press.

Jones, Margaret. 2000. "British Colonial Health Policy, 1900–1949: Ceylon and Asian Colonies." Ph.D. thesis, University of Bristol.

Jones, Margaret 2003. "Tuberculosis, housing and the colonial state: Hong Kong, 1900–1950." *Modern Asian Studies*, 37:3, July, pp. 653–682.

Kaufman, Joan. 2009. "Infectious disease challenges in China." In Charles W. Freeman III (ed.) *China's Capacity to Manage Infectious Diseases. Global Implications*. Washington, D.C.: Center for Strategic and International Studies, pp. 3–14.

King, Gordon. 1998. "An episode in the history of the university." In Clifford Matthews and Oswald Cheung, *Dispersal and Renewal: Hong Kong University During the War Years*. Hong Kong: Hong Kong University Press, pp. 85–103.

Kiple, Kenneth F. 1993. *The Cambridge World History of Human Disease*. Cambridge: Cambridge University Press.

Kuan, Hsin-chi. 1979. "Political stability and change in Hong Kong." *International Journal of Sociology*, 9:3, pp. 121–142.

Kuang, Zhiwen (Kwong Chi Man). 2015. *Chongguang zhilu: Riju Xianggang yu Taiping yang zhanzheng, 1942–1945* [Road to Liberation: Japanese Occupation of Hong Kong and the Pacific War, 1942–1945]. Hong Kong: Cosmos Books.

Kwong Chi Man and Tsoi Yiu Lun. 2014. *Eastern Fortress: A Military History of Hong Kong, 1840–1970*. Hong Kong: Hong Kong University Press.

Lam, T. P. 2001. "Strengths and weaknesses of traditional Chinese medicine and Western medicine in the eyes of some Hong Kong Chinese." *Journal of Epidemiology and Community Health*, 55:10, pp. 762–765.

Lau, Joseph T. F., H. Y.Tsui, and M. Phil. 2003. "Surveillance of discriminatory attitudes toward people living with HIV/AIDS among the general public in Hong Kong from 1994–2000." *Disability and Rehabilitation*, 25:24, pp. 1354–1360.

Lau, Joseph T. F., XilinYang, H. Y. Tsui, Ellie Pang. 2004. "SARS related preventive and risk behaviours practiced by Hong Kong-mainland China cross border travelers during the outbreak of SARS epidemic in Hong Kong." *Journal of Epidemiology and Community Health*, 58:12, pp. 988–996.

Lau, Siu Kai. 1982. *Society and Politics in Hong Kong*. Hong Kong: The Chinese University Press.

Lau, Stuart. 2013. "Mainland Chinese migrants since 1997 now make up 10pc. of Hong Kong population." *South China Morning Post*, 21 March.

Lau, Y. W. 2002. *A History of the Municipal Councils of Hong Kong 1883–1999: From the Sanitary Board to the Urban Council and the Regional Council*. Hong Kong: Leisure and Cultural Services Department.

Law, Kam-yee and Kim-ming Lee. 2006. "Citizenship, economy and social exclusion of mainland Chinese immigrants in Hong Kong." *Journal of Contemporary Asia*, 36:2, pp. 217–242.

Law, Yuen Han [Luo Wanxian]. 2007. "Xifang yixue yu zhimin guanzhi: yi erci shijie dazhan qian Xianggang he Xinjiapo wei bijiao gean" [Western Medicine and Colonial Rule: Pre-WWII Hong Kong and Singapore as Comparative Cases]. Ph.D. thesis, Hong Kong Baptist University.

Lee, Albert. 2003. "The need for integrated primary health care to enhance the effectiveness of health services." *Asia-Pacific Journal of Public Health*, 15:1, pp. 62–67.

Lee, Jik-Joen. 2009. *The Colonial Government of Hong Kong's Development of Social Welfare: From Economic and Social Service Perspectives*. Hong Kong: Department of Social Work, The Chinese University of Hong Kong.

Lee, Rance P. L. 1975. "Health services system in Hong Kong: professional stratification in a modernizing society." *Inquiry*, 12:2, Supplement, pp. 51–62.

Lee, Shiu-Hung. 1985. "Malaria in Hong Kong." *Journal of Society of Community Medicine*, 15:1, pp. 7–17.

Lee, Shiu-Hung et al. 1996. "Resurgence of cholera in Hong Kong." *Epidemiology and Infection*, 117:1, pp. 43–49.

Lee, Shiu-Hung. 1999. "Public health issues in Hong Kong and China." *Journal of Epidemiology and Community Health*, 53:3, pp. 130–131.

Lee, Shiu-Hung. 2003. "The SARS epidemic in Hong Kong: what lessons have we learned?" *Journal of the Royal Society of Medicine*, 96:8, pp. 374–378.

Lee, Shiu-Hung. 2003. "The SARS epidemic in Hong Kong." *Journal of Epidemiology and Community Health*, 57, pp. 652–654.

Lee, Yok-shiu F. 2002. "Tackling cross-border environmental problems in Hong Kong: initial responses and institutional constraints." *The China Quarterly*, 172, pp. 986–1009.

Leeming, Frank. 1975. "The earlier industrialization of Hong Kong." *Modern Asian Studies*, 9:3, pp. 337–342.

Leung, Angela Ki Che and Charlotte Furth (eds.). 2011. *Health and Hygiene in Chinese East Asia: Politics and Publics in the Long Twentieth Century*. Durham: Duke University Press.

Leung, W. T. 1983. "The new town programme." In T. N. Chiu and C. L. So (eds.) *A Geography of Hong Kong*. Hong Kong: Oxford University Press, pp. 210–217.

Levine, Phillippa. 2003. *Prostitution, Race, and Politics: Policing Venereal Disease in the British Empire*. New York: Routledge.

Levine, Phillippa. 1998. "Modernity, medicine and colonialism: the contagious disease ordinances in Hong Kong and the Straits Settlements." *Positions*, 6:3, pp. 675–705.

Li, C. K. 1981. "Epidemiology of malaria in the New Territories region, Hong Kong (1975–1980)." *Journal of the Hong Kong Society of Community Medicine*, 12:2, pp. 29–40.

Li, Shangren. 2012. *Diguo de yshi: Wanbade yu Yingguoredai yixue de chuangjian* [Physician of the empire: Manson and the creation of British tropical medicine]. Taibei: Yunchen wenhuashiye gufen youxian gongxi.

Li, Shu-fan. 1964. *Hong Kong Surgeon*. New York: E. P. Dutton & Co.

Lin, Oi-chu, William H. F.Kam, and Suk-yan Chan. 2004. "HIV/AIDS in Hong Kong. The emergence and impact of an epidemic." In Yichen Lu and Max Esses (eds.) *AIDS in Asia*. New York: Springer, pp. 145–151.

Liu, Shuyong. 1997. "Hong Kong: a survey of political and economic development over the past 150 years." *The China Quarterly*, 151, September, pp. 583–589.

Liu, Shuyong. 2009. *Jianming Xianggang shi* [A brief history of Hong Kong]. Hong Kong: Joint Publishing Co.

Liu, Zhipeng and Zhou Jiajian ed. 2009. *Tun sheng ren yu: Ri zhi shiqi Xianggang ren de ji ti hui yi* [The Tests of Endurance and Sufferance: An Oral Hisitory of Hong Kong People During the Japanese Occupation]. Hong Kong: Zhonghua Bookstore.

Lo, Danny. 1985. "Malaria stalks trail of tourists." *Hong Kong Standard*, April 8.

Loh, Christine and Civic Exchange. 2004. *At the Epicenter: Hong Kong and the SARS Outbreak*. Hong Kong: Hong Kong University Press.

Loh, Christine *et al.* 2011. "Hong Kong-Mainland Innovations in Environmental Protection since 1980." *Asian Survey*, 51:4, pp. 610–632.

Louis, Wm Roger. 1997. "Hong Kong: the critical phrase, 1945–1949." *The American Historical Review*, 102:4, pp. 1052–1084.

Ma, Qiusha. 1995. "The Rockefeller Foundation and modern medical education in China, 1915–1951." Ph.D. thesis, Case Western Reserve University.

MacKenback, J. P. 1994. "The epidemiologic transition theory." *Journal of Epidemiology and Community Health*, 48, pp. 329–332.

MacPherson, Kerrie L. 2001. "Health and empire: Britain's national campaign to combat venereal diseases in Shanghai, Hong Kong and Singapore." In R. Davidson *et al. Sex, Sin and Suffering: Venereal Disease and European Society since 1870*. London: Routledge, pp. 173–190.

MacPherson, Kerrie L. 2008. "One public, two health systems: Hong Kong and China integration without convergence." *China Review*, 8:1, pp. 85–104.

Martin, E. A. (ed.). 2010. *Concise Medical Dictionary*. 8th. Oxford: Oxford University Press.

Martin, Michael F. 2007. *CRS Report for Congress; Hong Kong. Ten Years after the Handover*. Washington, D.C.: Congressional Research Service.

Martin, R. M. 1846. *Reports, Minutes and Dispatches on the British Position and Prospects in China*. London: Harrison and Co. Printers.

Mcmenemey, W. H. 1973. "Medical History: The Lancet, 1823–1973." *British Medical Journal*, 5882 (September 29), pp. 680–684.

Meyer, David. 2008. "Structural changes in the economy of Hong Kong since 1997." *China Review*, 8:1, pp. 7–29.

Miners, Norman. 2002. "Industrial development in the colonial empire and the Imperial Economic Conference at Ottawa 1932." *The Journal of Imperial and Commonwealth History*, 30:2, pp. 53–76.

Moodie, A. S. 1962. "Tuberculosis in Hong Kong." *Tubercle*, 44, pp. 334–345.

Morley, Ian. 2007. "City chaos, contagion, and social justice." *Yale Journal of Biology and Medicine*, 80:2, pp. 61–72.

Morton, Brian. 1989. "Pollution of coastal waters of Hong Kong." *Marine Pollution Bulletin*, 20:7, pp. 310–318.

National Association for the Appeal of the Contagious Diseases Act. 1882. Lord Kimberley's Defence of the Government Brothel System at Hong Kong: Correspondence Relating to the Contagious Ordinances in Hong Kong.

Ng, Anthony. 1989. "Medical and health." In T. L. Tsim and Bernard H. K. Luk (eds.) *The Other Hong Kong Report 1989*. Hong Kong: The Chinese University Press, pp. 189–214.

Ng, Anthony. 1990. "Medical and Health." In Richard Y. C. Wong and Joseph Y. S. Cheng (eds.) *The Other Hong Kong Report 1990*. Hong Kong: The Chinese University Press, pp. 393–427.

Ng, Lun Ngai Ha. 1983. *Interactions of East and West: Development of Public Education in Early Hong Kong*. Hong Kong: The Chinese University Press.

Ngo, Tak-wing. 1996 "The East Asian Anomaly Revisited: The Politics of Laissez-faire in Hong Kong, 1945–1985." Ph.D. Thesis, University of London.

Ngo, Tak-wing. 1999. "Industrial history and the artifice of laissez-faire colonialism," In Ngo Tak-wing (ed.) *Hong Kong's History: State and Society under Colonial Rule*. London: Routledge, pp. 119–140.

Pattison, Stephen. 1992. "Vietnamese migrants in Hong Kong." *In Defense of the Alien*, 15, pp. 138–142.

Pekelharing, C. A. and C. Winkler. 1893. *Beriberi: Researches Concerning its Nature and Cause and the Means of its Arrest*. Trans. by James Cantlie. Edinburgh: Young H. Pentland.

Perry, Jane. 2004. "Two Hong Kong politicians resign in wake of SARS report," *British Medical Journal*, 329:7458 (July 17), p. 130.

Phillips, David R. 1988. *The Epidemiological Transition in Hong Kong: Changes in Health and Disease since the Nineteenth Century*. Hong Kong: Center of Asian Studies, University of Hong Kong.

Phillips, David R. 1994. "Epidemiological transition: implications for health and health care provision." *Geografiska Annaler. Series B. Human Geography*, 76:2, pp. 71–89.

Pryor, Edward G. 1975. "The great plague of Hong Kong." *Journal of the Hong Kong Branch of the Royal Asiatic Society*, 15, pp. 61–70.

Queen Elizabeth Hospital (comp.). 2013. *Yiyuanren.qing.shi – Yilishabai yiyuan wushizhounian koushu lishi* ["QEH – A People's history. An oral history for the golden jubilee of Queen Elizabeth Hospital"]. Hong Kong: Cognizance Publishing.

Rydings, H. A. 1973. "Transactions of the China Medico-Chirurgical Society, 1845–6." *Journal of the Hong Kong Branch of the Royal Asiatic Society*, 13, pp. 13–27.

SARS Expert Committee. 2003. *SARS in Hong Kong: from Experience to Action*. Hong Kong: Hong Kong Government.

Scott, Henry H. 1921. "The prevalence and character of tuberculosis in Hong Kong." *Annals of Tropical Medicine and Parasitology*, 15, p. 213.

Selwyn-Clarke, Selwyn. 1946. *Repors on the Medical and Health Conditions in Hong Kong for the Period 1st January 1942–31 August 1945*. London: HMSO.

Selwyn-Clarke, Selwyn. 1975. *Footprints: The Memoirs of Sir Selwyn Selwyn-Clarke*. Hong Kong: Sino-American Publishing Company.

Shen, Jianfa. 1997. "Population and migration trends in Hong Kong." *Geography*, 82:3, pp. 269–271.

Sims, L. D. *et al.* 2003. "Avian influenza in Hong Kong, 1997–2002." *Avian Diseases*, 47, pp. 832–838.

Sinn, Elizabeth. 1989. *Power and Charity: The Early Years of the Tung Wah Hospital*. Hong Kong: Oxford University Press.

Sinn, Elizabeth (ed.). 1990. *Between East and West: Aspects of Social and Political Development in Hong Kong*. Hong Kong: Centre of Asian Studies, University of Hong Kong.

Siu, Alan and Y. C. Richard Wong. 2004. "Economic impact of SARS: the case of Hong Kong." *Asian Economic Papers*, 3:1, pp. 62–83.

Smart, Alan. 2006. *The Shek Kip Mei Myth: Squatters Fire and Colonial Rule in Hong Kong, 1950–1963*. Hong Kong: Hong Kong University Press.

Smith, Carl T. 1995. "The first child labour law in Hong Kong." In *A Sense of History: Studies in the Social and Urban History of Hong Kong*. Hong Kong: Educational Publishing Company, pp. 213–239.

Snacken, Renee *et al.* 1999. "The next influenza pandemic: lessons from Hong Kong, 1997." *Emerging Infectious Diseases*, 5:2, pp. 195–203.

Snow, Philip. 2003. *The Fall of Hong Kong: Britain, China and the Japanese Occupation*. New Haven: Yale University Press.

Solomon, Tom. 1997. "Hong Kong, 1894: the role of James A. Lowson in the controversial discovery of the plague bacillus." *The Lancet*, 350, pp. 59–62.

Starling, Arthur *et al.* 2006. *Plague, SARS and the Story of Medicine in Hong Kong*. Hong Kong: Hong Kong University Press.

Sturm-Ramirez, Katharine M. *et al.* 2004. "Reemerging H5N1 influenza viruses in Hong Kong in 2002 are highly pathogenic to ducks," *Journal of Virology*, 78:9 (May), pp. 4892–4901.

Sung, Yun-Wing. 1997. "The Hong Kong economy through the 1997 barrier." *Asian Survey*, 37:8, pp. 705–719.

Sutphen, Mary P. 1995. "Imperial hygiene in Calcutta, Cape Town, and Hong Kong: The Early Years of Sir William John Richie Simpson (1855–1931)." Ph.D. Thesis, Yale University.

Sutphen, Mary P. 1997. "Not what, but where: bubonic plague and the reception of germ theories in Hong Kong and Calcutta, 1894–1897." *Journal of the History of Medicine and Allied Sciences*, 52:1, pp. 81–113.

Sutphen, Mary P. 1997. "Rumored power: Hong Kong, 1894 and Cape Town, 1901." In Andrew Cunnigham and Bridie Andrews (eds.) *Western Medicine as Contested Knowledge*. Manchester: Manchester University Press, pp. 241–261.

Tang, Kwong-leung. 1998. *Colonial State and Social Policy: Social Welfare Development in Hong Kong, 1842–1997*. Lanham: University Press of America.

Taylor, Gwen. 2002. "Hong Kong's health care reform: nursing an ailing health care system back to life." *Perspective on Business and Economics*. 20, pp. 1–23.

Taylor, W. R. J. 1999. "Measles in Vietnamese refugee children in Hong Kong." *Epidemiology and Infection*, 122:3, pp. 441–446.

"The Basic Law of the Hong Kong Special Administration Region of the People's Republic of China." 1988. Reprinted in Hungdah Chiu (ed.) *The Draft Basic Law of Hong Kong: Analysis and Documents*. Baltimore: University of Maryland School of Law, pp. 117–143.

The Friends of China and Hong Kong Gazette, 5 October 1843.

Ticozzi, Sergio. 1997. *Historical Documents of the Hong Kong Catholic Church*. Hong Kong: Hong Kong Catholic Diocesan Archives.

Tsang, Steve. 1995. *A Documentary History of Hong Kong: Government and Politics*. Hong Kong: Hong Kong University Press.

Tsang, Steve. 1997. "Government and politics in Hong Kong: a colonial paradox." In Judith M. Brown and Rosemary Foot (eds.) *Hong Kong's Transitions, 1842–1997*. London: MacMillan Press, pp. 62–83.

Tsang, Steve. 2004. *A Modern History of Hong Kong*. London: I. B. Tauris.

Ure, Gavin. 2012. *Governors, Politics, and the Colonial Office: Public Policy in Hong Kong, 1918–1958*. Hong Kong: Hong Kong University Press.

Vaughan, T. D. and D. J. Dwyer. 1966. "Some aspects of postwar population growth in Hong Kong." *Economic Geography*, 42:1, pp. 37–51.

Wang, Jeanette. 2015. "HIV/AIDS still largely a taboo subject in Hong Kong and much of East Asia." *South China Morning Post*, March 23.

Wellington, A. R. 1937. *Memorandum regarding changes in the public health organization of Hong Kong during the period 1929 to 1937* (No. 4 of Sessional Papers for the Year of 1937). Hong Kong: Hong Kong Government.

Welsh, Frank. 1997. *A History of Hong Kong*. London: HarperCollins.

Wong, Frances K. Y. 1998. "Health care reform and the transformation of nursing in Hong Kong." *Journal of Advanced Nursing*, 28:3, pp. 473–482.

Wong, Hung. 2005. "The quality of life of Hong Kong poor household in the 1990s: levels of expenditure, income security and poverty." *Social Indicators Research*, 71:1/3, pp. 411–440.

Wong Richard Y. C. and Joseph Y. S. Cheng (eds.). 1990. *The Other Hong Kong Report 1990*. Hong Kong: The Chinese University Press, pp. 393–427.

Wong, Timothy Man Kong. 2003. "The changing meanings of governorship in Hong Kong between 1946 and 1997, with reference to the China factor in Hong Kong." *Hong Kong Journal of Modern Chinese History*, 1, pp. 113–130.

Wong, Timothy Man Kong. 2006. "Local voluntarism: the medical mission of the London Missionary Society in nineteenth century China." In David Hardiman (ed.) *Healing Bodies, Saving Souls: Medical Missions in Asia and Africa*. Amsterdam: Rodopi, pp. 87–113.

Wong, Timothy Man Kong. 2008. "Institutional changes, research culture, and professionalism: development of medical sciences in Hong Kong in the 1980s." *Journal of Comparative Asian Development*, 7:2, pp. 285–309.

Wong, Timothy Man Kong. 2009. "Higher education and research culture in Hong Kong: with special reference to medical education, research, and professionalism, 1880s-1980s." In Ricardo Mak (ed.) *Transmitting the Ideal of Enlightenment: Chinese Universities since the Nineteenth Century*. Lanham: University Press of America, pp. 83–108.

Wong, Ting-Hong. 2002. *Hegemonies Compared: State Formation and Chinese School Politics in Postwar Singapore and Hong Kong*. New York: Routledge.

Wong, Tze Wai *et al.* 1995. "Prevalence and determinants of the use of traditional Chinese medicine in Hong Kong." *Asia Pacific Journal of Public Health*, 8:3, pp. 167–170.

Wong, Tze Wai *et al.* 1999. "Air pollution and hospital admissions for respiratory and cardiovascular diseases in Hong Kong." *Occupational and Environmental Medicine*, 56:10, pp. 679–683.

Wong, Tze Wai *et al.* 2002. "Associations between daily mortalities from respiratory and cardiovascular diseases and air pollution in Hong Kong, China." *Occupational and Environmental Medicine*, 59:1, pp. 30–35.

Wong, Victor C. W. 1999. *The Political Economy of Health Care Development and Reform in Hong Kong*. Aldershop: Ashgate.

Woo, J. *et al.* 1997. "An estimate of chronic disease burden and some economic consequences among the elderly Hong Kong population." *Journal of Epidemiology and Community Health*, 51, pp. 486–489.

Working Party on Government Policies and Practices. 1963. *Report of the 1963 Working Party on Government Policies and Practices with Regards to Squatters, Resettlement and Government Low Coast Housing*. Hong Kong: The Working Party.

World Health Organization (WHO) and Department of Health, Hong Kong. 2012. *Health Service Delivery Profile: Hong Kong (China)*. Manila: Western Pacific Region WHO.

Xie, Yong Guang. 1995. *Sannian ling bage yue de kunan* [Hardships and Sufferings during the Three Years and Eight Months]. 2nd. Hong Kong: Ming Pao Publishing Company.

Xie, Yong Guang. 1998. *Xianggang zhongyi yao shi hua* [History of Chinese medicine and pharmacology in Hong Kong]. Hong Kong: Sanlian Shudian.

Yanghe Yiyuan Lishi, 1922–2012 [History of the Hong Kong Sanatorium & Hospital, 1922–2012]. Hong Kong: Hong Kong Sanatorium & Hospital.

Yep, Ray. 2008. "The 1967 riots in Hong Kong: the diplomatic and domestic fronts of the colonial governor." *The China Quarterly*, 193, pp. 122–139.

Yeung, Linda. 2013. "Hong Kong urgently needs a hospital to teach traditional Chinese medicine." *South China Morning Post*. December 16.

Yip, Ka-che. 2009. *Disease, Colonialism, and the State: Malaria in Modern East Asian History*. Hong Kong: Hong Kong University Press.

Yip, Ka-che. 2009 "Colonialism, Disease, and Public Health: Malaria in the History of Hong Kong." In Ka-che Yip ed., *Disease, Colonialism, and the State: Malaria in Modern East Asian History*. Hong Kong: Hong Kong University Press.

Yip, Ka-che. 2009. "Revolution and Enlightenment: The Rise of Biomedical Education in China, 1910–1950." In Ricardo Mak (ed.) *Transmitting the Ideal of Enlightenment: Chinese Universities since the Nineteenth Century*. Lanham: University Press of America, pp. 67–82.

Yip, Ka-che. 2012. "Science, culture, and disease control in colonial Hong Kong." In Liping Bu, Darwin H. Stapleton, and Ka-che Yip (eds.) *Science, Public Health and the State in Modern Asia*. London: Routledge, pp.15–32.

Yip, Ka-che. 2012. "Segregation, isolation, and quarantine: protecting Hong Kong from Diseases in the pre-war period." *Journal of Contemporary Asian Development*, 11:1, pp. 93–116.

Yip, Ka-che. 2012. "Health care in a harmonious society: crises and challenges in post-1978 China." In Joseph Tse-Hei Lee *et al.* (eds.) *China's Rise to Power: Conception of State Governance*. New York: Palgrave Macmillan, pp. 181–206.

Yip, Ka-che. 2015. "Transition to decolonization: the search for a health policy in post-war Hong Kong, 1945–1985." In Liping Bu and Ka-che Yip (eds.) *Public Health and National Reconstruction in Post-war Asia: International Influences, Local Transformations*. New York: Routledge, pp. 13–33.

Yuen, Peter P. 1992. "Medical and health," In J. Y. S. Cheng (ed.) *The Other Hong Kong Report 1992*. Hong Kong: The Chinese University Press, pp. 279–296.

Yuen, Richard M. F. 2014. "The challenge of an ageing society from a health care perspective." *Public Administration and Policy*, Spring, pp. 1–14.

Zhao, Xiaobin et al.2004. "Income inequalities under economic restructuring in Hong Kong." *Asian Survey*, 44:3, pp. 442–473.

Zhang, Jiawei (Cheung Ka-wai). 2000. *Xianggong 67 baodong neijing* [The inside story of the 1967 riot in Hong Kong]. Hong Kong: Pacific Century Press.

Zheng, Hongtai (Victor Cheng) and Huang Shaolun (Wong Siu-lun). 2005. *Xianggang Miye Shi* [A History of Rice Trade in Hong Kong]. Hong Kong: Joint Publishing Co.

Zietz, Bjorn P. and Hartmut Dunkelberg. 2004. "The history of the plague and the research on the causative agent *Yersinia Pestis.*" *International Journal of Hygiene and Environmental Health*, 207, pp. 165–178.

Index

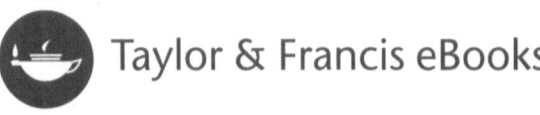
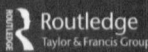